THE
CALORIE,
CARBOHYDRATE,
AND **CHOLESTEROL**
DIRECTORY

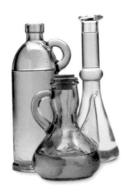

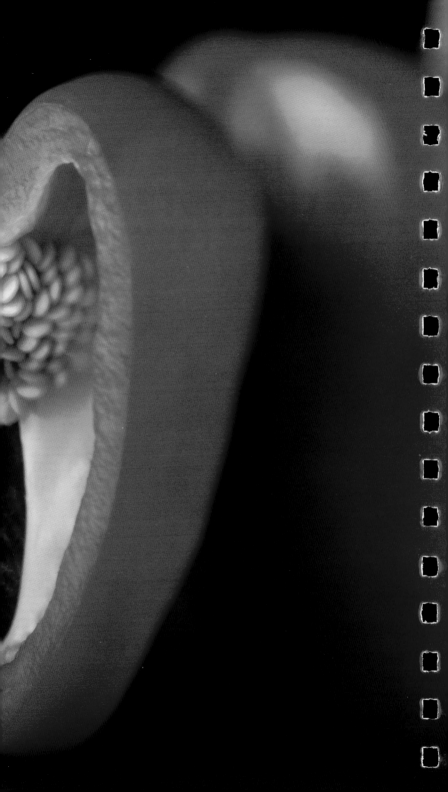

THE
CALORIE,
CARBOHYDRATE,
AND CHOLESTEROL
DIRECTORY

Nutritional facts and figures
for hundreds of everyday foods

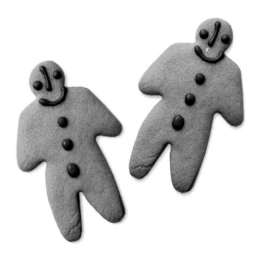

Martha Schueneman

Text and design copyright © The Ivy Press Limited 2004

First published in the UK in 2004 for Grange Books
an imprint of Grange Books plc
The Grange
Kingsnorth Industrial Estate
Hoo, nr Rochester
Kent ME3 9ND
www.Grangebooks.co.uk

by arrangement with THE IVY PRESS LIMITED

ISBN: 1-84013-665-0

Note from the publisher
Information given in this book is not intended to be
taken as a replacement for medical advice. Any person
with a condition requiring medical attention should
consult a qualified medical practitioner or therapist.

This book was conceived, designed, and produced by
THE IVY PRESS LIMITED
The Old Candlemakers
Lewes, East Sussex BN7 2NZ

Creative Director: PETER BRIDGEWATER
Publisher: SOPHIE COLLINS
Editorial Director: STEVE LUCK
Senior Project Editor: CAROLINE EARLE
Design Manager: TONY SEDDON
Designer: JANE LANAWAY
Consultant Nutritionist: ROBIN KLINE MS, RD, CCP
Picture Research: SHARON DORTENZIO, ANNA DAVIES
Additional Photography: IAN PARSONS

Printed and bound in China

Contents

Introduction

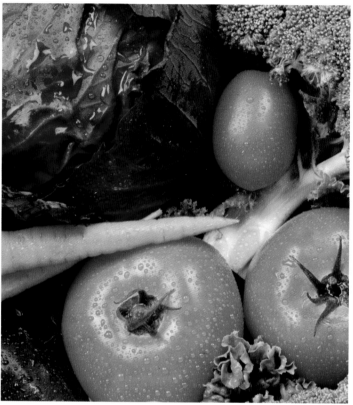

Fresh vegetables are a valuable source of nutrients.

Nutrition is dynamic. As new discoveries are made, what's touted as a miracle food one day is found to have little or no effect on health the next. How do you evaluate the conflicting messages and sort through the hype?

There's no easy path, but knowing a little bit about what foods are made of is a good place to start.

CALORIES COUNT

Fast food, junk food, soda, too many calories, too much fat, too many carbs, and too little exercise have all been blamed for the growing obesity epidemic. Which is it? The short answer is it can be all of the above.

Foods are made up of fats, carbohydrates, and protein. Fats weigh in at 9 calories per gram. Protein and carbohydrates have 4 calories per gram (alcohol contains 7 calories per gram).

Different people need different amounts of calories. Larger and more active people need more calories than do smaller, less active people. Depending on size, age, and activity level, an adult woman typically needs about 1,700–2,000 calories a day; the typical adult man needs 2,000–2,500. As you grow older, your metabolism slows down and you require fewer calories. If you've been slowly gaining weight over the years, but haven't changed your eating habits or exercise routine, it's because you're eating more calories than you need to at this point in your life.

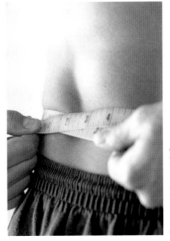

Are you gaining weight?

Ice cream

If you eat more calories than you burn off, you'll gain weight. If you eat fewer calories than you burn off, you'll lose weight.

A pound of fat is about the same as 3,500 calories, so to lose one pound a week, you must either cut 500 calories from the amount you eat every day or increase your exercise to burn off 500 calories a day, or do both.

Because fat contains more calories by weight than protein or carbohydrate, it makes sense to limit the amount of fat you eat, but this can backfire. Fat is more satisfying and helps to make you feel full longer. If you're constantly hungry but avoid fat, you may increase the amount of carbohydrates in your diet, and end up eating the same number of calories.

But there's more to good nutrition and healthy eating than just calories. Will you lose a pound a week if you eat 1,200 calories a day in ice cream and potato chips? If you require 1,700 calories a day, yes, you will. Will you be able to maintain your health on such a diet? In a word, no.

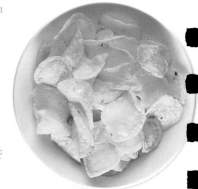

Potato chips

For good health, you need a variety of nutrient-dense foods. Deeply colored vegetables and fruits, lean meats and fish, dairy, whole grains, nuts, and some fats qualify. White bread and foods made from refined grains, sugary foods, most packaged and convenience foods, and foods high in some fats don't.

Tomato

Does that mean that you should never eat a doughnut? No. But if you eat them several times a week, you are probably not getting the nutrients you need. Your mother was right—if you fill up on snacks, you won't eat your dinner. To put it another way, if you fill up on foods high in refined sugar and refined flours and trans fats, which often are low in vitamins and minerals, you'll eat fewer nutrient-rich foods.

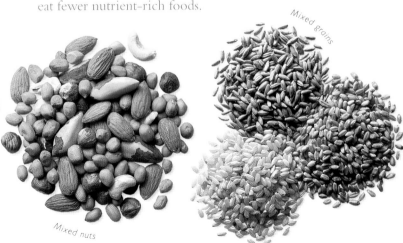

Mixed grains

Mixed nuts

THE SKINNY ON FAT AND CHOLESTEROL

Fat and cholesterol have bad reputations, so it may come as a surprise to learn that both are essential to good health. Both perform an array of vital functions.

Fat cushions organs, helps regulate body temperature, and can help control your appetite. Not all types of fat are good for you, however.

Cholesterol is not a fat; it has no calories. It is a waxy lipid, or fatlike substance, that exists in every cell in your body. It is used to make the sheaths that protect nerves and to make certain hormones, including testosterone and estrogen. The liver manufactures all that your body needs—about 1,000 milligrams a day. Lipoproteins carry cholesterol from the liver throughout the body via the bloodstream.

There are several types of lipoproteins, but two of the most significant in terms of heart disease are LDL, or low-density lipoprotein (often called "bad" cholesterol), and HDL, or high-density lipoprotein (the "good" one). LDL isn't very efficient. As it moves through the bloodstream, it "drops" cholesterol, which can build up on artery walls. This buildup causes arteries to harden and narrow, a condition called atherosclerosis. HDL picks up this dropped cholesterol and carries it back to the liver. If you have a lot of LDL in your blood, you increase the risk for atherosclerosis and heart disease. If you have high HDL levels, your risk may be lower.

So how do you lower cholesterol levels? Many things affect cholesterol levels, including whether you smoke and how much you exercise, and what you eat influences it as well. This may seem counterintuitive, but avoiding foods high in cholesterol doesn't necessarily decrease the amount of cholesterol in your blood.

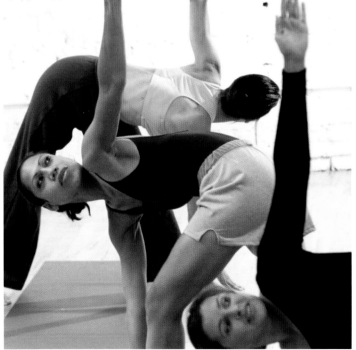

Regular exercise will help to lower cholesterol levels.

Butter

For years, saturated fats—they're the ones that are solid at room temperature, like butter— were thought to be the main culprit. Saturated fats raise blood cholesterol levels, so people were cautioned to cut down on meat, butter, and dairy products, which all contain varying amounts of saturated fat. In the last few years, however, it's been discovered that saturated fats raise both LDL and HDL levels, so although your blood has more LDLs depositing cholesterol on artery walls, it also has more HDLs picking them up. The negative effects are lessened.

There are fats even more dangerous than saturated fats— trans fats. Trans fats are made by incorporating hydrogen into liquid vegetable oils so that they become solid or semisolid at room temperature. Any "hydrogenated vegetable oil" or "partially hydrogenated vegetable oil" is a trans fat. Trans fats increase LDL levels and lower HDL levels. As a result, your blood has more LDLs dropping cholesterol, but fewer HDLs to bring it back to the liver.

If you eat a lot of fried foods, packaged snack foods like chips, packaged baked goods like cookies and crackers and cakes, or anything made with vegetable shortening, you're eating a lot of trans fats. What's alarming is that many of the foods that are so high in this killer fat are labeled to let you believe they are good for you—they're cholesterol-free and have no saturated fats!

SWEETS FOR THE SWEET

There's another fatal flaw in the typical American diet: it's heavily weighted toward refined carbohydrates.

Like fats, there are good and bad carbohydrates. Those in vegetables, whole grains, nuts, legumes, and fruits come with fiber that slows down the speed at which they are digested, as well as with a vast array of vitamins, minerals, and compounds that affect the health in beneficial ways. Carbohydrates from refined grains and sugars—white bread, pasta, crackers, soda, chips, and cookies, for example—are low in natural nutrients and fiber.

Whole-wheat crackers

Carrots

Refined carbohydrates cause blood sugar to shoot up rapidly, then plummet a short while later. Limiting the amount of refined carbohydrates in your diet can regulate your blood sugar levels, reducing the risk of diabetes, hypertension, and even food cravings. The glycemic index (GI) measures how rapidly 50 grams of carbohydrate from a food—not 50 grams of a food—raise blood sugar levels compared to 50 grams of glucose. Glucose is given a value of 100, and the GI of other foods is a percentage. Carrots, for example, have a high glycemic index. If you eat 50 grams of carbohydrate from carrots, then your blood sugar levels will increase 71 percent compared to eating 50 grams of carbohydrate from sugar. However, you'd have to eat about 1½ pounds of carrots to get 50 grams of carbohydrate, far more than the typical half-cup serving. Fifty grams of carbohydrate from a bagel will increase your blood sugar 72 percent compared to eating 50 grams of sugar. One bagel can have as much as 70 grams of carbohydrate, so it will have a far more dramatic effect on your blood sugar levels than carrots will, despite the two foods' similar GI values.

Testing foods for their GI value is complicated. As a result, very few foods have been tested. Most of those that have are available in Australia and England, and their recipes and formulas are often different from U.S. ones. Also, you can't assume that similar foods have similar GIs. For instance, the amount of fiber can slow down the rate at which sugar is absorbed—oatmeal cookies (which are fairly high in fiber) have a fairly low glycemic index value and high-fat, low-fiber vanilla wafers have a high GI.

The most reputable and up-to-date sources have been used for the GI values listed in this book, but there simply isn't enough reliable research to include values for all foods. In addition, many public health groups and organizations are divided on the GI's usefulness as a tool in determining a food's nutritional value. Should you avoid foods that have a high GI? Not necessarily—carrots

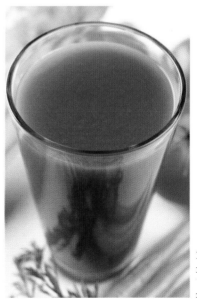

Vegetable juice

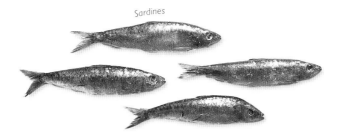

Sardines

contain plenty of nutrients that you need. A good rule of
thumb is to limit foods that contain a lot of refined sugar
and little else in the way of nutrients.

WHAT EATING HEALTHFULLY MEANS

So how do you put this all together? Should you count
calories, limit fat, or limit carbohydrates? What's the balance
between protein, carbohydrate, and fat that you should
seek for good health?

Look at the Food Guide Pyramid or a traditional nutrition
book, and you'll probably be told to eat a limited amount of
fat—no more than 30 percent of your calories every day—
and to make sure that 55–60 percent of your calories come
from carbohydrate, and 10–15 percent come from protein.

If you've limited your fat intake for the past several years
and have still gained weight, you will know that low fat is
only part of the picture. When foods are processed to remove
fat, sugar is often added. The fat content may be lower, but

the carbohydrate content is higher and the number of calories may be the same. Fat, you may have learned, is not the enemy—at least not all fats. Eating fat doesn't make you fat—in fact, eating foods high in fat can help you to eat less overall, because fat can satisfy you. Anyone who's eaten way too many fat-free cookies and still feels hungry knows this.

1 percent milk

But carbohydrates aren't necessarily the enemy either—vegetables, legumes, fruits, and grains are high in carbohydrate. They're also high in vitamins, minerals, and phytochemicals (compounds that occur naturally in plants). Thousands of phytochemicals have been identified, but only a few hundred have been studied. Most appear to have antioxidant

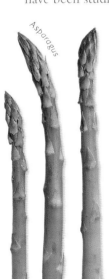

Asparagus

properties—that is, they dispose of potentially harmful oxygen by-products—and are believed to protect from diseases as different as high cholesterol and the eye disorder macular degeneration.

Plant foods also supply fiber. Although fiber contains no nutrients, it can lower

cholesterol and reduce the risk
of heart disease, stabilize blood
sugar levels, and promote a
healthy digestive tract.

Pretzels

Eating a diet that's high in trans fats and in refined carbohydrates, however, can be particularly hazardous to your health. Instead, eat foods that have been minimally processed—choose plain brown rice, cooked in broth and mixed with herbs or spices, rather than a package of white rice with a seasoning packet; plain yogurt topped with blueberries rather than a container of blueberry yogurt; whole-wheat toast with apple butter rather than an apple

Plain chips

turnover; or shrimp sautéed with garlic in olive oil, rather than breaded and deep-fried shrimp. You'll get more vitamins and nutrients, and minimize your intake of sugar, salt and trans fats.

Also, eat foods in moderation. A handful of chips at a Superbowl party or a picnic won't hasten your demise, but a 3-ounce bag of chips every day at lunch can have a pronounced negative effect on your weight and health.

RECOMMENDED DIETARY GUIDELINES

As scientists learn more about food and how our bodies use it, dietary guidelines change. In fact, the USDA is considering revising its Food Pyramid. The balance of macronutrients—protein, fat, and carbohydrate—may change, but savvy food choices include opting for those that are high in beneficial fats (particularly monounsaturated and polyunsaturated fats), complex carbohydrates, and lean sources of protein over those that are high in harmful fats (especially trans fats), refined carbs, and fatty sources of protein. You'll find the skinny about them in this book. Most nutrition experts and food scientists agree that it's wise to adhere to the following daily limits:

Calories—women	1700–2,000 calories
Calories—men	2,000–2,500 calories
Cholesterol	300mg
Sodium	2,400mg
Fiber	at least 20mg

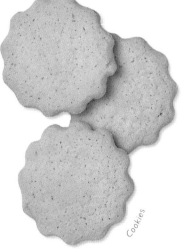

Cookies

NUTRIENT DATA

Most of the nutrition information in this book is from the USDA National Nutrient Database for Standard Reference, Releases 15 and 16. The USDA doesn't always include sugars in its analysis. Because sugars are a type of carbohydrate, the grams of sugars in a food will never be more than the grams of carbohydrate. When specific brands or foods are mentioned, the nutrient data comes from the company's Web site.

THE CALORIE, CARBOHYDRATE, AND CHOLESTEROL DIRECTORY

How to use this book

The Calorie, Carbohydrate, and Cholesterol Directory packs a lot into every page: breakdowns of vital nutrients in charts and bullets, as well as information on what to look for when shopping and how to prepare food for maximum flavor and nutrition.

CHARTS

● The nutrient amounts are for recommended portion sizes (e.g., for meats), or for common portion sizes (e.g., for fruits). In most instances, the nutrient information came from the USDA's Nutrient Data Web site. If data for a particular nutrient are not available but the food may contain that nutrient, "NA" is used. "NA" is also used if the food probably affects blood sugar levels but the glycemic index is not available for it. If the food doesn't have an effect on blood sugar levels, a "0" appears in the GI column.

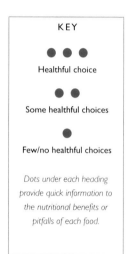

KEY

● ● ●
Healthful choice

● ●
Some healthful choices

●
Few/no healthful choices

Dots under each heading provide quick information to the nutritional benefits or pitfalls of each food.

STYLE 1 cup cooked	CALORIES	CHOLESTEROL mg	SODIUM mg	TOTAL FAT g	SATURATED FAT g
Cornmeal (polenta)	110	0	11	1.1	0.2
Grits, quick cooking	145	0	0	0.5	tr
Millet	207	0	3	1.7	0.3
Quinoa	159	0	9	2.5	0.3
Buckwheat groats	155	0	7	1	tr

110

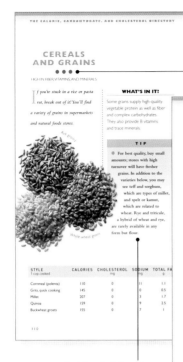

The key on the facing page explains the dots. Use these for at-a-glance information for each category.

THE CALORIE, CARBOHYDRATE, AND CHOLESTEROL DIRECTORY

CEREALS AND GRAINS
● ● ● ●
HIGH IN FIBER, VITAMINS, AND MINERALS

If you're stuck in a rice or pasta rut, break out of it! You'll find a variety of grains in supermarkets and natural foods stores.

WHAT'S IN IT!
Some grains supply high-quality vegetable protein as well as fiber and complex carbohydrates. They also provide B vitamins and trace minerals.

TIP
● For best quality, buy small amounts; stores with high turnover will have fresher grains. In addition to the varieties below, you may see teff and sorghum, which are types of millet, and spelt or kamut, which are related to wheat. Rye and triticale, a hybrid of wheat and rye, are rarely available in any form but flour.

STARCHY FOODS

Millet

WHAT'S THE BEST!
● Whole grains are digested slowly and have less of an effect on blood sugar levels than processed and refined grains.

WHAT'S NOT SO GOOD!
● Be wary of buying grains sold in clear containers. Exposure to heat or sunlight can cause nutrient loss.

STYLE 1 cup cooked	CALORIES	CHOLESTEROL mg	SODIUM mg	TOTAL FA
Cornmeal (polenta)	110	0	11	1.1
Grits, quick cooking	145	0	0	0.5
Millet	207	0	3	1.7
Quinoa	159	0	9	2.5
Buckwheat groats	155	0	7	1

110

SATURATED FAT g	PROTEIN g	CARBOHYDRATE g	FIBER g	SUGARS g	GI
0.2	1	23	2.2	0	NA
tr	3	31	0.5	0.2	NA
0.3	6	41	2.2	0.7	NA
0.3	6	29	2.5	NA	NA
tr	6	33	4.5	2.2	L

111

Look here for information about buying, cooking, and storing foods, or about specific information for a particular food.

If you're wondering whether a food is good for you —or want to know how you can make it part of a healthful diet—look here.

Not sure how to tell kale from collards or quinoa from cornmeal? Photographs of different foods appear on every spread.

PROTEIN g	CARBOHYDRATE g	FIBER g	SUGARS g	GI
	23	2.2	0	NA
	31	0.5	0.2	NA
6	41	2.2	0.7	NA
6	29	2.5	NA	NA
6	33	4.5	2.2	L

111

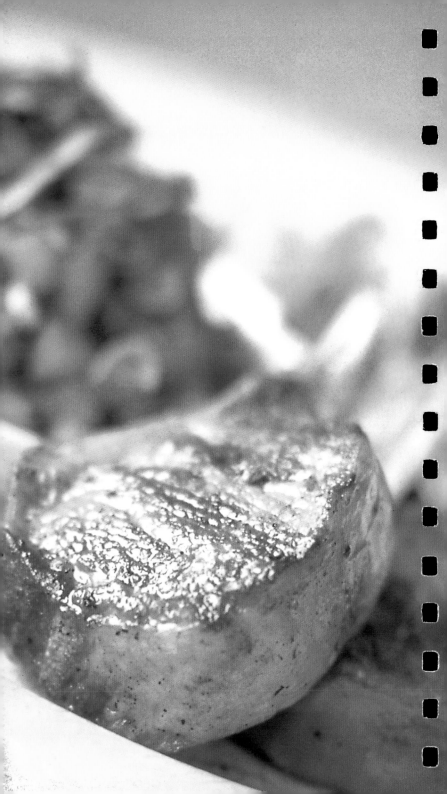

MEAT AND GAME

*Perennial favorites beef and pork, and
processed meats like bacon and sausage are not
"heart-healthy" in and of themselves, but they can
be part of a balanced diet. Three rules will help
you remain healthy while enjoying them:*

- *Trim all external fat before cooking;*
- *Limit portions to 3 oz of cooked meat;
  this is about the size of a deck
  of cards, or the palm of your hand;*
- *Consume these foods in moderation.
  Eating bacon a few times a month is one thing,
  a few times a week is something else entirely.*

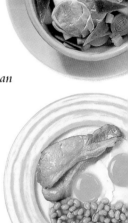

*The nutrition charts in this section
assume that meat is trimmed of all visible
external fat before cooking. Serving sizes
are 3 oz, unless noted. To end up
with 3 oz of cooked meat, start with a
4-oz boneless cut or an 8-oz bone-in cut.*

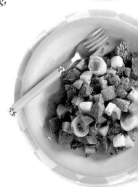

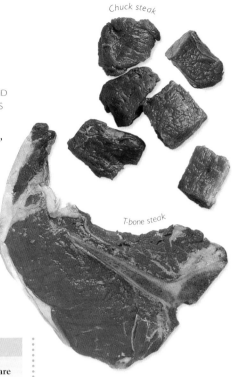

Chuck steak

BEEF

● ●

GOOD SOURCE OF PROTEIN AND
IRON. HIGH IN SATURATED FATS

*Beef is high in protein, iron,
and vitamin B12, but
despite these nutrients, treat
this red meat with caution—
it's high in cholesterol
and saturated fat, even when
external fat is trimmed.*

T-bone steak

TIP

● Brisket and shoulder cuts are
better braised or pot-roasted in
liquid. Make them a day ahead
and chill them. The fat will
congeal on the top of the sauce
and can be scraped off.

WHAT'S IN IT?

A 3-oz serving of beef, cooked with
about 1/8 inch of external fat contains
about 75mg cholesterol. Remove the
fat before cooking and you can cut
that by up to one third.

STYLE 3-oz	CALORIES	CHOLESTEROL mg	SODIUM mg	TOTAL FAT g
T-bone steak, broiled	168	48	60	8.2
Porterhouse, broiled	180	53	59	9.5
Tip round, roasted	150	69	55	5
Chuck roast	179	90	56	6.5
Ground beef (90% lean)	173	70	64	9
Ground beef (85% lean)	197	73	67	11.9
Ground beef (80% lean)	209	73	71	13.6

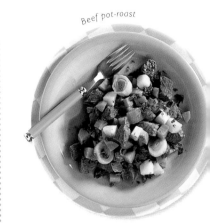

Beef pot-roast

WHAT'S THE BEST?

◉ Lean cuts have little marbling, or fat within the muscles. They can be tough, though, and are better braised.

◉ Clever cooking. Broiling and grilling steaks allow fat to drain off. If you do fry, do so without added oils.

WHAT'S NOT SO GOOD?

◉ Big servings. Keep your portions small—don't eat a serving that's larger than the size of a deck of cards.

◉ Expensive cuts. Avoid them— most contain much more fat. Exceptions: lean ground beef and tenderloin.

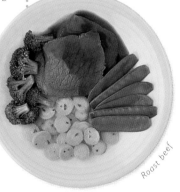

Roast beef

You can enjoy beef as part of a balanced diet, but trim off all visible external fat. Pot-roasting is an ideal cooking method for tough cuts of beef.

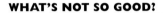

SATURATED FAT g	PROTEIN g	CARBOHYDRATE g	FIBER g	SUGARS g	GI
2.8	22	0	0	0	0
3.3	22	0	0	0	0
1.8	24	0	0	0	0
2.3	28	0	0	0	0
3.7	21	0	0	0	0
4.7	21	0	0	0	0
5.3	20	0	0	0	0

VEAL

● ●

HIGH IN PROTEIN AND B VITAMINS

Veal has earned a bad reputation recently due to the way calves are raised. If you can get past that, it's a nutritional bargain, especially compared to beef and lamb. Veal is lower in fat and calories, but slightly higher in cholesterol.

TIPS

● Veal has little marbling (fat inside the muscle), so it's best sautéed in a small amount of oil or braised.

● Cuts from the shoulder and lower part of the leg tend to be tough; they are best braised or stewed.

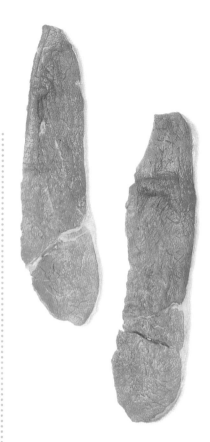

WHAT'S IN IT?

A 3-oz veal cutlet contains more cholesterol than the same size serving of ground beef, but has about one fifth as much saturated fat.

STYLE 3-oz	CALORIES	CHOLESTEROL mg	SODIUM mg	TOTAL FAT g
Cutlet (top round)	156	91	65	3.9
Stewing veal	160	124	80	3.7
Rib roast	151	98	83	6.3
Shank	151	107	80	3.7
Loin roast	149	90	82	5.9
Ground veal	146	88	71	6.4

WHAT'S THE BEST?

● Ground veal has much less fat than ground beef; it usually comes from the leg or shoulder.

● Cuts from the upper part of the leg, such as cutlets or scallops, are the leanest.

WHAT'S NOT SO GOOD?

● Most recipes. Veal is low in fat, but is often dipped in breadcrumbs before frying, or covered with cheese and rich sauces. Instead, dredge it in a little flour before sautéing, and serve it with a lemony or wine-based sauce.

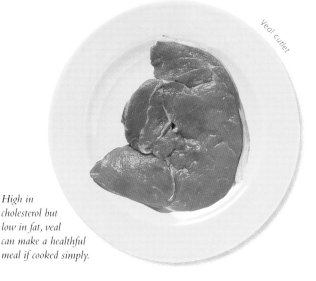

Veal cutlet

High in cholesterol but low in fat, veal can make a healthful meal if cooked simply.

SATURATED FAT g	PROTEIN g	CARBOHYDRATE g	FIBER g	SUGARS g	GI
1.1	28	0	0	0	0
1.1	30	0	0	0	0
1.8	22	0	0	0	0
0.9	17	0	0	0	0
2.2	24	0	0	0	0
2.6	21	0	0	0	0

LAMB

● ●

HIGH IN PROTEIN, IRON,
AND ZINC. SIMILAR TO BEEF IN
FAT AND CHOLESTEROL

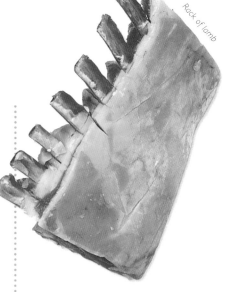

Rack of lamb

*L*amb is raised to be consistently lean and tender today, but choose cuts carefully—some can be exceedingly high in fat. The fat is easy to trim off and lessens the fat content and lamb's gamy flavor.

Lamb cutlets

TIP

● Trimming off as much of the external fat as possible cuts down on the cholesterol but won't eliminate it. That's because cholesterol is in the lean tissue or muscle, not just in the fat.

STYLE 3-oz	CALORIES	CHOLESTEROL mg	SODIUM mg	TOTAL FAT g
Leg, roast	162	76	58	6.6
Rib roast	197	75	69	11.3
Shoulder	237	103	65	12
Ground lamb	240	82	69	16.7
Loin, roast	172	74	56	8.3

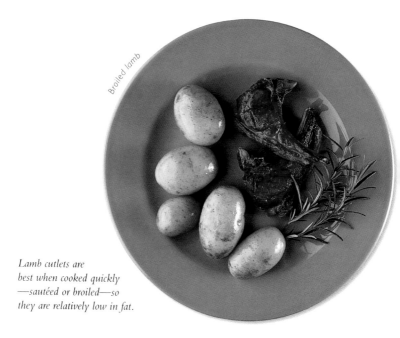

Broiled lamb

Lamb cutlets are best when cooked quickly —sautéed or broiled—so they are relatively low in fat.

WHAT'S IN IT?

● A 3-oz serving of leg of lamb provides several B vitamins, but about one third of the recommended daily allotment of cholesterol.

WHAT'S THE BEST?

● Shank is the leanest cut, but it can be tough. It's best braised or stewed. Roast well-trimmed lamb on a rack so the fat can drip away.

WHAT'S NOT SO GOOD?

● Older lamb. Recognized by its dark red color, this has a very strong flavor and more marbling. Instead, look for lamb with pink to deep pink meat and pearly white fat.

● Packaged ground lamb can get more than 60 percent of its calories from fat. Choose lean cuts from the leg, trim all external fat, and grind it yourself or have the butcher grind it.

SATURATED FAT g	PROTEIN g	CARBOHYDRATE g	FIBER g	SUGARS g	GI
2.3	24	0	0	0	0
4	22	0	0	0	0
4.3	30	0	0	0	0
6.9	21	0	0	0	0
3.2	23	0	0	0	0

PORK
● ●

AMONG THE LEANEST MEAT AVAILABLE.
SOME CUTS ARE VERY FATTY

Pork today is up to 30 percent leaner than it was 20 years ago—but you must choose wisely, because some pork is among the fattiest meat. Very lean pork can be tricky to cook—it can become dry and tough.

WHAT'S IN IT?

A 3-oz serving of pork tenderloin supplies just 1.4g saturated fat and 67mg cholesterol. The same size serving of spareribs weighs in at 9.4g saturated fat and 103mg cholesterol.

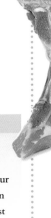

pork chops

TIP

● If you eat a lot of chicken as a low-fat protein, consider using boneless pork loin in your recipes instead. Pork tenderloin is comparable to chicken breast in nutrition.

STYLE 3-oz	CALORIES	CHOLESTEROL mg	SODIUM mg	TOTAL FAT g
Spareribs	337	103	79	26
Ground pork	252	80	62	17.7
Picnic shoulder, braised	211	97	87	11
Center loin chop, pan-fried	190	60	44	10
Tenderloin, roast	139	67	48	4.1
Fresh ham (pork leg), roasted	183	78	55	9

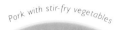
Pork with stir-fry vegetables

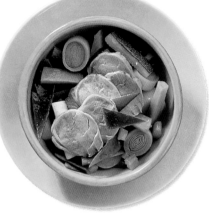

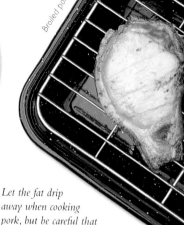
Broiled pork chop

Choose lean cuts and cook them with plenty of vegetables to make pork a low-fat meal.

Let the fat drip away when cooking pork, but be careful that the meat does not dry out.

WHAT'S THE BEST?

● Loin cuts—center loin and tenderloin—are leanest, but they can be pricey. Buy a whole loin and cut it into chops, then freeze. Be sure to cut off the external fat before cooking.

● Clever cooking. Roast on a rack or grill so the fat drips away. Slice boneless loin cuts into strips for stir-fried dishes with lots of vegetables.

WHAT'S NOT SO GOOD?

● Rib cuts. Country-style ribs and spareribs get about 70 percent of their calories from fat!

● Careless cooking. Pork doesn't require a lot of attention, but it can dry out if it is overcooked. But make sure that you don't undercook it either. It should have an internal temperature of 160°F.

SATURATED FAT g	PROTEIN g	CARBOHYDRATE g	FIBER g	SUGARS g	GI
9.5	25	0	0	0	0
6.5	22	0	0	0	0
3.5	27	0	0	0	0
3.7	24	0	0	0	0
1.4	24	0	0	0	0
3.1	24	0	0	0	0

VARIETY MEATS

●

EXCELLENT SOURCE OF VITAMINS
AND MINERALS
CAN BE VERY HIGH IN CHOLESTEROL

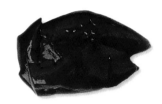

Liver

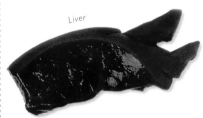

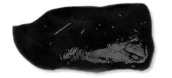

*L*iver is the most common variety meat. Unlike most meat, it is extremely high in vitamins A and C, as well as iron, zinc, and vitamin B12. Sweetbreads (the thymus of calves or lamb) are one of the few animal foods that supply vitamin C.

TIP

● Cook these foods carefully—they can toughen quickly, as anyone who was forced to eat liver and onions as a child remembers. Look for recipes in recently published cookbooks.

WHAT'S IN IT?

A 3-oz serving of beef liver supplies 409mg cholesterol—109mg more than the recommended intake for an entire day—and about seven times the vitamin A for the day. In general, variety meats are rich in iron and trace minerals like copper, zinc, and phosphorus, and in B vitamins.

STYLE 3-oz	CALORIES	CHOLESTEROL mg	SODIUM mg	TOTAL FAT g
Calves' liver, pan-fried	208	281	112	9.7
Beef liver, pan-fried	184.5	409	90	6.8
Tongue	240.5	91	51	18
Sweetbreads (veal)	148	398	56	3.6
Pigs' feet	165	85	25.5	10.5
Tripe (3½ oz)	91	157	68	4

WHAT'S THE BEST?

● Calves' liver is more tender than beef liver, and it has a milder flavor. It's fairly high in cholesterol, but it's significantly lower than beef liver.

● Sweetbreads are considered a delicacy; they are comparatively low in calories and are quite low in saturated fat.

WHAT'S NOT SO GOOD?

● Organ meats in general are highly perishable and must be stored and handled carefully. Plan to cook them the day you purchase them.

● Pesticides, fertilizers, antibiotics, and other chemicals can accumulate in an animal's liver. Seek out this organ from a younger animal, or from organically raised cattle.

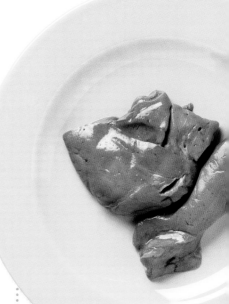

Liver is high in vitamins and minerals, but cook liver carefully—it's best eaten lightly sautéed.

SATURATED FAT g	PROTEIN g	CARBOHYDRATE g	FIBER g	SUGARS g	GI
3.6	25	0	0	0	0
2.3	23	0	0	0	0
7.6	19	0	0	0	0
1.2	27	0	0	0	0
3.6	16	0	0	0	0
1.4	12	2	0	0	0

PRESERVED AND PROCESSED MEATS

●

CURED PRODUCTS ARE HIGH-FAT AND HIGH-SODIUM

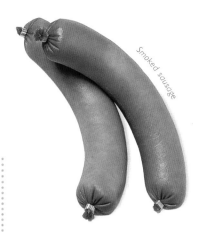

Smoked sausage

*P*rocessed meats are almost always high in fat and cholesterol. They include organs and very fatty scraps. Sodium is often used to cure and flavor meats.

WHAT'S IN IT?

A 3-oz serving of extra-lean ham has only 45mg cholesterol and 4.5g fat, but it has more than 1,000mg sodium, almost half the recommended daily allowance.

TIP

● Pay careful attention to serving sizes. Most bacon and sausage Nutrition Facts labels specify a serving as 1 or 2 oz—that's about 1 slice of bacon or about a 1–2-inch length of kielbasa.

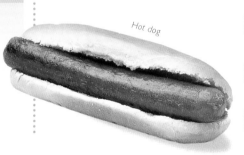

Hot dog

STYLE 3-oz, unless noted	CALORIES	CHOLESTEROL mg	SODIUM mg	TOTAL FAT g
Turkey bacon (14g)	35	13	170	2.8
Bacon (3 slices)	109	16	303	9.4
Canadian bacon (2 slices)	87	27	727	4
Hot dog (1)	135	22	504	12.4
Italian sausage	125	25	478	7
Cured ham (regular)	151	50	1275	7.7
Cured ham (extra-lean)	123	45	1023	4.7
Beef bologna (1 slice)	89	18	330	8.1

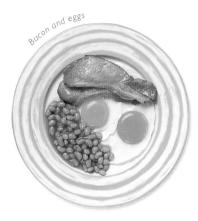

Bacon and eggs

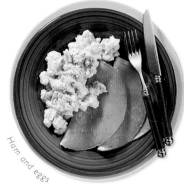

Ham and eggs

Bacon is high in sodium and in fat. Save it for special-occasion breakfasts and brunches.

It may be a lean option, but check out the sodium content for cured ham. It's best used sparingly as a flavoring for soups and casseroles.

WHAT'S THE BEST?

● Look for low-sodium, low-fat alternatives like turkey bacon. Extra-lean ham must contain no more than 5 percent fat by weight.

● Clever cooking—baked bacon. Set bacon slices on a rack so that the fat can drain off, then bake at 350°F until crispy.

WHAT'S NOT SO GOOD?

● Cured hams and dry and semi-dry sausages may have been cured with sodium nitrate or sodium nitrite.

● Big portions. Use preserved and processed meats as flavorings, not entrées. Add a bit of smoky sausage to a soup, or crumble a small amount of bacon onto a salad.

SATURATED FAT g	PROTEIN g	CARBOHYDRATE g	FIBER g	SUGARS g	GI
0.7	2	0.2	0.2	0	0
3.3	6	0.1	0	0	0
1.3	11	0.6	0	0	0
4.8	6	0.6	1	0	0
2.7	14	2	0	0	0
2.7	19	0	0	0	0
1.5	18	1	0	0	0
3	4	0.7	0.4	0	0

VENISON

● ● ●

VERY LOW IN SATURATED FAT

*A*n excellent alternative for red-meat lovers, venison is leaner than beef. Ranch-raised venison is less gamy and more tender than venison from the wild, though some connoisseurs believe that farm-raised deer meat tastes bland when compared to the meat of wild animals.

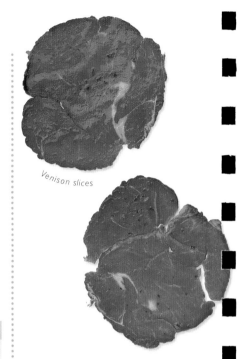

Venison slices

TIP

● Venison can toughen quickly and must be cooked carefully, although the best techniques differ for the various cuts. Consult a game cookbook for best results.

WHAT'S IN IT?

Venison is a superb source of lean protein. It also supplies generous amounts of vitamin B12 and iron, as well as riboflavin, niacin, and zinc. A 3-oz serving contains just 3g of total fat.

STYLE 3-oz	CALORIES	CHOLESTEROL mg	SODIUM mg	TOTAL FAT g
Top round steak	129	72	38	1.6
Shoulder roast	162	96	44	3.4
Ground venison, pan-broiled	159	83	66	7

WHAT'S THE BEST?

● Good cuts. All are low in fat and contain similar amounts of cholesterol.

● Because venison has so little fat, it must be cooked carefully. Cuts from the shoulder, rump, and leg tend to be tough. Braise or stew these, or grind them to make burgers.

WHAT'S NOT SO GOOD?

● What fat there is usually has a very gamy flavor. Cutting it off lowers the fat and reduces the strong taste.

If you like red meat, venison is one of the most healthful choices because it is low in saturated fat.

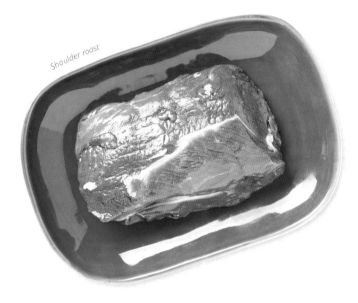

Shoulder roast

SATURATED FAT g	PROTEIN g	CARBOHYDRATE g	FIBER g	SUGARS g	GI
0.8	27	0	0	0	0
1.7	31	0	0	0	0
3.4	22	0	0	0	0

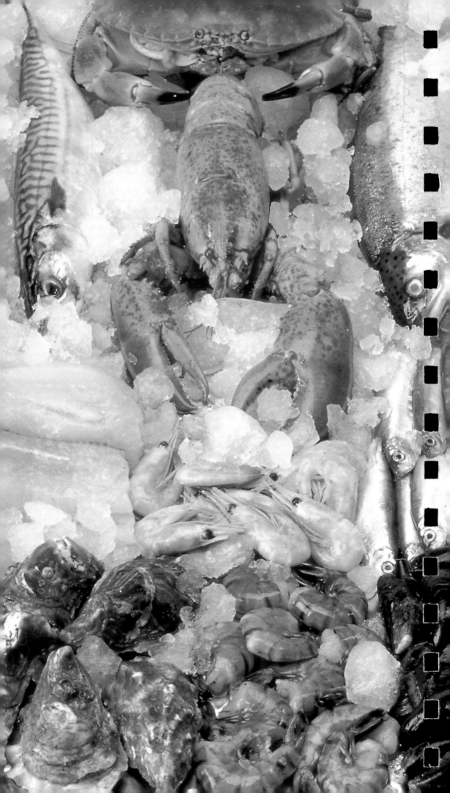

FISH, SHELLFISH, AND POULTRY

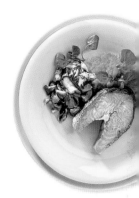

If you're looking to reduce the amount of fat in your diet but don't want to sacrifice flavor, you'll find a wealth of options among fish and shellfish, as well as among the tremendous variety of poultry.

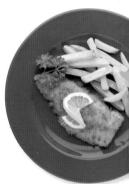

Fish, particularly cold-water fatty fish such as salmon, mackerel, and sardines, is an excellent source of omega-3 fatty acids. This is a type of polyunsaturated fat that can guard against heart disease and hypertension, and can reduce levels of triglycerides (a lipid, or fatty substance).

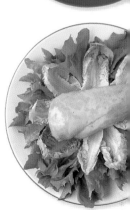

If you can't face yet another chicken breast, consider other cuts or other birds. Even birds that you might think are high in fat are in line with chicken once you remove the skin.

Baked salmon

FATTY FISH

● ● ●

FULL OF BENEFICIAL FATS
HEART-HEALTHY

*F*atty (or oily) fish is an excellent source of protein and B vitamins, but be selective. Some fish are more nutritious than others, and large fish can harbor toxins.

Low in saturated fats, salmon also contains omega-3 fatty acids, which are essential to healthy cell function.

TIP

● Limit consumption of large ocean fish (such as swordfish, shark, and tuna) to 12 oz per week. Because they feed on other fish, they can accumulate high levels of mercury.

Salmon steak

WHAT'S IN IT?

All fatty fish are low in saturated fats, fairly low in cholesterol, and are a good source of omega-3 essential fatty acids. They're called "fatty" because they are more than 5 percent fat by weight.

STYLE 3-oz, unless noted	CALORIES	CHOLESTEROL mg	SODIUM mg	TOTAL FAT g
Salmon (farmed)	175	54	52	10.5
Salmon (wild)	155	60	48	7
Sardines, canned* (2)	50	34	121	2.7
Anchovies (5)	42	17	734	2
Canned* tuna, albacore	109	36	320	2.5
Canned* tuna, light	99	26	287	0.7
Fresh tuna, grilled	118	49	40	1
Swordfish	132	43	98	4.4

* water-packed

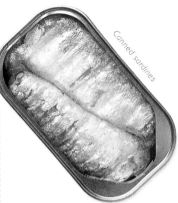

Canned sardines

WHAT'S THE BEST?

● All fatty fish contain some omega-3 fats, but Atlantic salmon is among the varieties containing the highest amounts.

● Fresh tuna has a meaty texture that makes it a heart-healthy alternative to beef.

Canned sardines are an excellent source of calcium, but drain off all surplus oil before use.

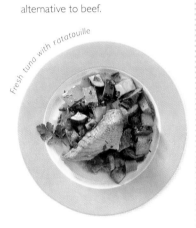

Fresh tuna with ratatouille

Fresh tuna's meaty texture makes it a good choice for people who don't like fish.

WHAT'S NOT SO GOOD?

● Canned fish can be very high in sodium, but sardines and salmon can also be rich in calcium.

● To reduce oil from oil-packed canned fish, and to reduce sodium levels, dump canned fish in a colander and rinse; drain well before using.

SATURATED FAT g	PROTEIN g	CARBOHYDRATE g	FIBER g	SUGARS g	GI
2.1	19	0	0	0	0
1	22	0	0	0	0
0.4	6	0	0	0	0
0.4	6	0	0	0	0
0.6	30	0	0	0	0
0.2	22	0	0	0	0
0.3	26	0	0	0	0
1.2	22	0	0	0	0

WHITE FISH

● ● ●

VERY LOW IN FAT

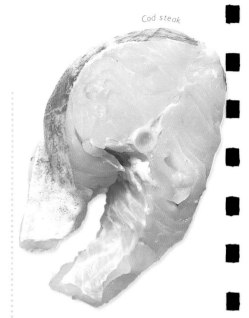

Cod steak

Often sold as fillets, white-fleshed fish is very lean and cooks quickly—it's ideal for hectic weeknights. Fillets tend to be thin and delicate, so they're often breaded before cooking—the coating makes them less fragile. Often dipping fillets in seasoned flour is sufficient to protect them.

TIP

● Don't cook fish in a microwave. Because fish fillets are so thin and cook so fast, there's a chance they won't get hot enough to kill any microorganisms.

WHAT'S IN IT?

Hundreds of species of saltwater and freshwater fish are available. In general, most are low in fat, calories, and cholesterol and are high in B vitamins; some are high in vitamins A, D, and E. Steer clear of processed fish, such as fishsticks—they're high in trans fats and preservatives.

STYLE 3-oz	CALORIES	CHOLESTEROL mg	SODIUM mg	TOTAL FAT g
Flounder and Sole	99	58	89	1.3
Cod	89	47	66	0.7
Perch	99	97	67	1
Catfish	129	54	68	7
Trout	162	63	57	7
Fishsticks (1)	76	31	163	3.4

WHAT'S THE BEST?

⬤ White fish are all very low in fat. Most are mild in flavor and are often interchangeable in recipes—ask your fishmonger which is the freshest.

⬤ Don't turn up your nose at frozen fish. If it was properly frozen at sea, it can be higher in quality than fresh fish.

WHAT'S NOT SO GOOD?

⬤ Processed fish. Batter-dipped, breaded, and deep-fried fish is high in fat, particularly trans fats.

⬤ Chemicals. Fish can harbor PCBs, mercury, and other toxins. If you catch your own fish, check with local authorities to make sure it is safe to eat.

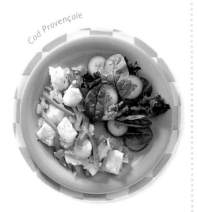

Cod Provençale

A very healthful choice, white fish is low in fat, high in vitamins, and quick to cook.

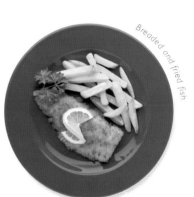

Breaded and fried fish

Coated in batter or breading and fried, even the leanest fish becomes high in fat.

SATURATED FAT g	PROTEIN g	CARBOHYDRATE g	FIBER g	SUGARS g	GI
0.3	21	0	0	0	0
0.1	19	0	0	0	0
0.2	21	0	0	0	0
1.5	16	0	0	0	0
1.3	23	0	0	0	0
0.8	4	6.6	0	0	0

SHELLFISH

● ● ●

VERY LOW IN SATURATED FAT

*S*hellfish includes crustaceans *(shrimp, lobster, crabs) and mollusks (clams, scallops, mussels, squid, octopus). All are low in calories and saturated fat and high in vitamins and minerals, though some are high in cholesterol and should be avoided by those who are sensitive to the effects of dietary cholesterol.*

WHAT'S IN IT?

Shellfish can be high in cholesterol, but research shows that the cholesterol in foods has less of an impact on blood cholesterol levels than does the saturated fat in food.

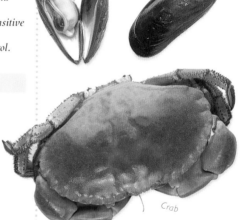

Mussels

Crab

TIP

● Shellfish is incredibly perishable. Plan to cook it the day you buy it, or buy frozen shellfish and put it in the freezer immediately when you get home.

STYLE 3-oz	CALORIES	CHOLESTEROL mg	SODIUM mg	TOTAL FAT g
Lobster	83	61	323	0.5
Shrimp	83	166	190	0.9
Scallops	75	28	137	0.6
Calamari, fried	149	221	260	6.4
Clams, steamed	126	57	95	1.7
Crabs, steamed	74	116	82	1.1
Mussels, steamed	146	48	314	3.8

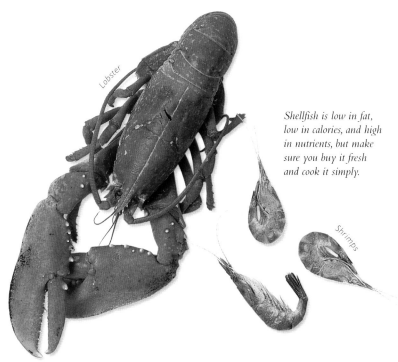

Lobster

Shrimps

Shellfish is low in fat, low in calories, and high in nutrients, but make sure you buy it fresh and cook it simply.

WHAT'S THE BEST?

● Scallops and lobster are almost fat-free and are very low in cholesterol. Shrimp are marginally higher in fat and significantly higher in cholesterol, and are rich in vitamin D.

● Smart cooking. Steam, grill, or sauté in olive oil. Shrimp and scallops are good for kebabs.

WHAT'S NOT SO GOOD?

● Shellfish is naturally low in calories, but this doesn't necessarily mean that all shellfish is good for you! Steer clear of fried shrimp, clams, and calamari.

● Skip the drawn butter and tartar sauces on your shellfish—cocktail sauce is the leaner choice.

SATURATED FAT g	PROTEIN g	CARBOHYDRATE g	FIBER g	SUGARS g	GI
0.1	17	0	0	0	0
0.2	17	0	0	0	0
0.07	14	2	0	NA	NA
1.6	15	7	0	NA	0
0.2	22	4	0	NA	0
0.2	15	0	0	0	0
0.7	20	6	0	NA	0

CHICKEN

● ●

GOOD SOURCE OF PROTEIN
CAN BE LOW IN SATURATED FAT

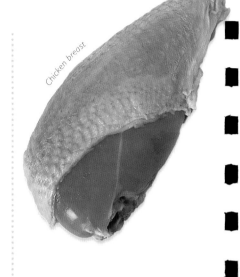

Chicken breast

Versatile, flavorful chicken is comparable to beef in the quality and quantity of its protein, yet can have a fraction of beef's fat. Chicken is also high in several B vitamins and in minerals like zinc and phosphorus.

TIP

● Before roasting a whole chicken or bone-in breasts, gently lift the skin off the meat and rub seasonings—an herb paste like pesto, or whole sage leaves or thyme sprigs—directly onto the flesh. You'll add flavor to the meat, not the skin.

WHAT'S IN IT?

Ounce for ounce, white meat chicken is lower in calories, fat, saturated fat, and cholesterol than dark meat; it's also slightly higher in protein and considerably higher in niacin.
Dark meat chicken contains more riboflavin, iron, selenium, and zinc.

STYLE 1 piece serving	CALORIES	CHOLESTEROL mg	SODIUM mg	TOTAL FAT g
Breast, w/o skin, roast	142	73	64	3
Breast with skin, roast	193	82	70	7.6
Thigh, w/o skin, roast	109	49	46	5.6
Thigh, with skin, roast	153	58	52	9.6
Drumstick, w/skin, roast	112	47	47	5.8
Cornish Game Hens	116	91	68	3.3

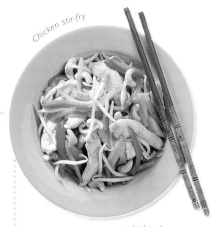
Chicken stir-fry

WHAT'S THE BEST?

● Smart cooking. Chicken takes
well to just about any cooking
method, so bake, roast, stir-fry, grill,
broil, or sauté it, or add it to
casseroles, soups, or salads.

● Skinless chicken breast. The
ubiquitous chicken breast gets
less than 20 percent of its
calories from fat.

WHAT'S NOT SO GOOD?

● Chicken skin. Keep the skin on
when you cook chicken to help keep
the meat moist, but remove it—and
any fat—before serving.

● Chicken wings. With very little
meat and a comparatively large
amount of skin, chicken wings get
62 percent of their calories from fat.

*Stir-fry chicken with lots of
vegetables for a super-nutritious
meal. Remove the skin to reduce
calories, fat, and cholesterol.*

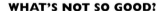
Skinless chicken breast

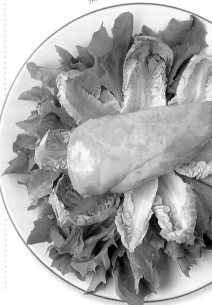

SATURATED FAT g	PROTEIN g	CARBOHYDRATE g	FIBER g	SUGARS g	GI
0.9	27	0	0	0	0
2.1	29	0	0	0	0
1.6	13	0	0	0	0
2.7	16	0	0	0	0
1.6	14	0	0	0	0
0.8	20	0	0	0	0

TURKEY

● ● ●

CAN BE LOW IN FAT AND
SATURATED FAT. EXCELLENT SOURCE
OF PROTEIN AND B VITAMINS

Not long ago it was hard to find turkeys most of the year, but now whole birds and turkey parts are widely available year round. Look for whole breasts or breast cutlets as alternatives to chicken.

WHAT'S IN IT?

Skinless turkey breast is the leanest meat of all. It has slightly more than half a gram of total fat in a 3-oz serving.

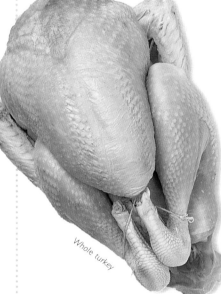

Whole turkey

TIPS

● Like chicken, turkey will be more moist and flavorful if you cook it with the skin on, then remove the skin before eating.

● Toms are slightly lower in fat and cholesterol than hens— but the difference is fairly small. Choose your holiday bird on the basis of how many people you are serving.

STYLE 3-oz	CALORIES	CHOLESTEROL mg	SODIUM mg	TOTAL FAT g
Breast, w/o skin roasted	115	71	44	0.6
Thigh, w/o skin, roast	138	95	67	3.7
Thigh, pre-basted	157	62	437	8.5
Ground	193	84	88	10.8

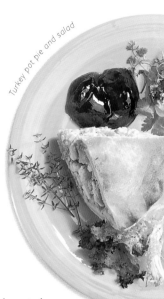

Turkey pot pie and salad

WHAT'S THE BEST?

● Ultra-low-fat turkey breast. Counteract any blandness by cooking with lots of fresh herbs and spices. Serve with savory, high-flavor sauces rather than high-fat gravy.

● Dressing baked out of the bird. Stuffing cooked in the bird can absorb fat, and there's a risk it won't become hot enough to kill bacteria. Play it safe and bake it separately.

Breast is leanest when it comes to turkey, though dark meat is still fairly lean. Use small amounts in pot pies.

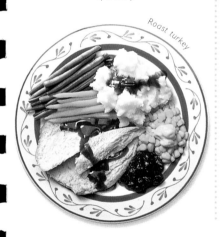

Roast turkey

WHAT'S NOT SO GOOD?

● Ground turkey. Often marketed as a low-fat alternative to ground beef, ground turkey is often made of higher-fat dark meat and skin. To be sure, have a butcher grind breast meat for you.

● Prebasted turkeys. A high-sodium solution is injected into the bird.

SATURATED FAT g	PROTEIN g	CARBOHYDRATE g	FIBER g	SUGARS g	GI
0.2	26	0	0	0	0
1.2	25	0	0	0	0
2.7	19	0	0	0	0
2.8	22	0	0	0	0

DUCK

● ●

CAN BE LOW IN FAT AND
SATURATED FAT

D uck has a reputation for being high in fat, but guess what? Once the skin is removed, duck breast is lower in total fat and saturated fat than chicken breast.

WHAT'S IN IT?

Duck is entirely dark meat poultry. A 3-oz portion of skinless duck breast provides nearly half of the RDA of niacin, iron, and selenium, and it's a good source of lean protein, too.

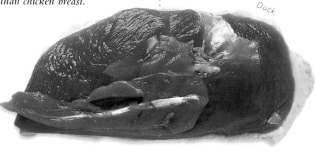

Duck

TIPS

● Duck contains comparatively little meat for the amount of bone that it contains: a 3–4-pound duck will feed around two to three people. Seek out duck breast, which has a higher meat-to-bone ratio.

● Unsure how to cook or serve duck? This richly flavored bird has more in common with beef and dark-meat chicken. Replace the steak in your favorite recipe with duck breast, or try using duck breast in chicken recipes instead.

STYLE 3-oz	CALORIES	CHOLESTEROL mg	SODIUM mg	TOTAL FAT g
Breast w/o skin, broiled	119	121	89	2.1
Breast w/skin, roasted	171	116	71	9.2
Leg, w/o skin, braised	151	89	92	5

WHAT'S THE BEST?

● As with other poultry, skinless duck is lower in fat and calories than duck with the skin still on.

● Smart cooking. Roasting whole duck is labor-intensive, because the skin is very fatty and grease accumulates rapidly in the pan. It's much easier to grill or broil duck breasts.

WHAT'S NOT SO GOOD?

● As with chicken fat, most duck fat is in or near the skin. Be sure to remove the skin before eating.

● Most duck sold in markets is frozen. Avoid any packages that have holes or are leaking (a sign that the birds have been mishandled), and adhere to any sell-by or use-by dates.

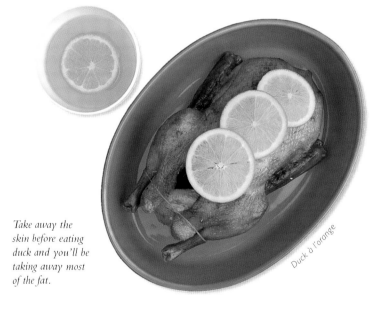

Duck à l'orange

Take away the skin before eating duck and you'll be taking away most of the fat.

SATURATED FAT g	PROTEIN g	CARBOHYDRATE g	FIBER g	SUGARS g	GI
0.4	23	0	0	0	0
2.5	21	0	0	0	0
1.1	25	0	0	0	0

GOOSE

●

HIGH IN FAT AND SATURATED FAT

*M*oist and succulent, goose makes for an impressive holiday feast. This bird is quite high in fat, even without the skin.

WHAT'S IN IT?

Roasted goose eaten without its skin has about 96mg cholesterol—almost one third of the recommended daily limit—and about one third of the recommended amount of saturated fat.

TIP

● Serve goose with tart sauces and side dishes to counteract its richness. Try unsweetened applesauce or a compote made of pears or dried fruits.

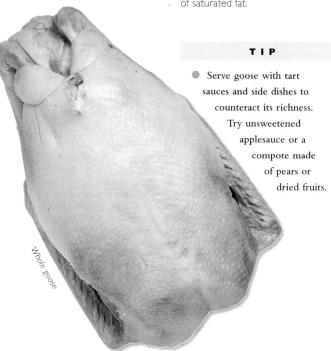

Whole goose

STYLE 3½-oz	CALORIES	CHOLESTEROL mg	SODIUM mg	TOTAL FAT g
Roast, w/skin	305	91	70	22
Roast, w/o skin	238	96	76	13

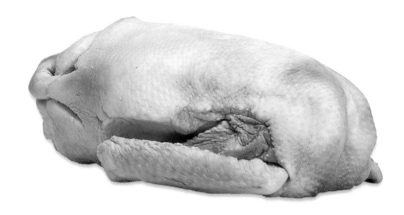

Goose is a high-fat, high-cholesterol bird,
so keep it for special occasions.

WHAT'S THE BEST?

● Smart cooking. Goose should be roasted. Make shallow slits in the skin of the breast to allow fat to drain off. Some cookbooks recommend roasting the bird breast-side down on a rack until almost done, then turning over to brown. Put a bit of water in the pan to keep the drippings from igniting. Don't broil goose—its fat could catch fire.

● Goose supplies generous amounts of B vitamins, as well as iron, selenium, and zinc.

WHAT'S NOT SO GOOD?

● Goose is a dark meat, and even with the skin removed is comparable to fattier cuts of beef.

● Fatty side dishes. Because goose is so rich, keep the accompaniments light. Rice pilaf, cooked in broth and studded with toasted almonds and golden raisins, is a good choice.

● As goose roasts, the fat will accumulate in the bottom of the pan. Check frequently and remove the excess (a turkey baster is an ideal tool).

SATURATED FAT g	PROTEIN g	CARBOHYDRATE g	FIBER g	SUGARS g	GI
6.9	25	0	0	0	0
4.6	29	0	0	0	0

GAME BIRDS

● ●

MOST ARE VERY LOW IN FAT
AND SATURATED FAT

arm-raised pheasant, quail, squab, and even ostrich can be found in most butchers and even some supermarkets. They tend to be specialty items and may be available seasonally, although larger markets may stock them (often with the frozen food) year round.

Quail

WHAT'S IN IT?

Game birds are almost all uniformly low in calories, fat, and cholesterol, and are high in protein, iron, and B vitamins.

TIPS

● Small birds within each species will be younger and more tender; some cooks believe that hens are more flavorful than males.

● Domestic game birds tend to be fattier and milder in flavor than wild birds—though compared to turkey and chicken, it is quite lean and can have a pronounced taste.

● Most game birds are small, so their yields are not the same as for chicken. A pheasant might serve about two people— and two quails will serve one.

STYLE 3½-oz	CALORIES	CHOLESTEROL mg	SODIUM mg	TOTAL FAT g
Pheasant	133	66	37	3.6
Quail	134	70	51	4.5
Squab	142	90	51	7.5
Ostrich leg	140	73	83	2

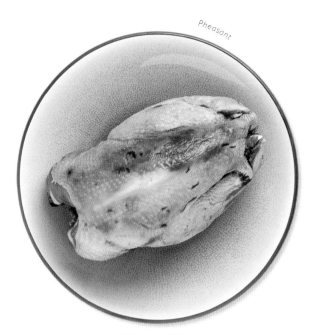

Pheasant

*Most game birds are
low in fat, but pheasant
is particularly lean.*

WHAT'S THE BEST?

● Ostrich and pheasant are the leanest choices. Ostrich is a dark red meat, similar to very lean beef.

● Smart cooking. The best techniques vary from one bird to another. Roasting and stewing are the most common methods of cooking.

WHAT'S NOT SO GOOD?

● Barding. Game birds tend to be so lean that some recipes instruct you to bard, or cover the birds (or their breasts) with bacon before roasting. This will keep them moist but ups the calorie, fat, and cholesterol content.

SATURATED FAT g	PROTEIN g	CARBOHYDRATE g	FIBER g	SUGARS g	GI
1.2	24	0	0	0	0
2.3	22	0	0	0	0
2	18	0	0	0	0
0.7	29	0	0	0	0

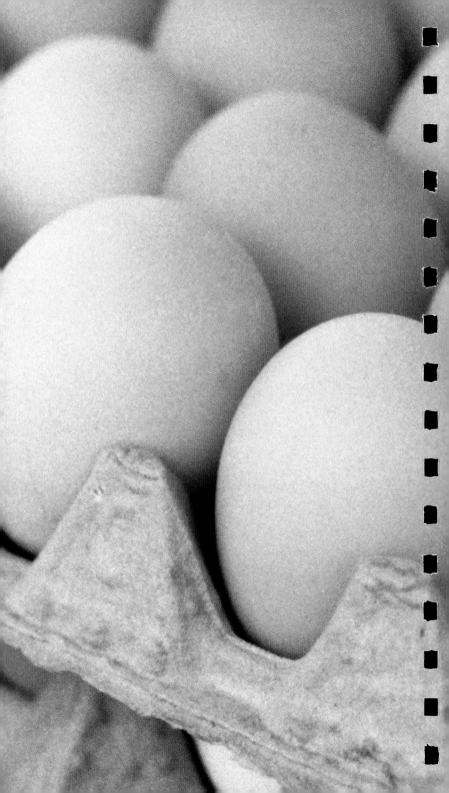

DAIRY FOODS AND EGGS

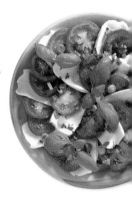

You might be tempted to eliminate dairy and eggs from your diet—after all, they're high in cholesterol and fat—but don't. Instead, just make smart choices.

Milk is an excellent source of calcium, as well as protein, zinc, vitamins A, B12, and D, and riboflavin. Cheese and yogurt contain similar nutrients in varying amounts; low-fat and fat-free varieties of dairy products abound and are worth investigating.

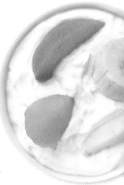

Eggs do indeed supply more than two thirds of the recommended daily limit of cholesterol, but they also contain every essential nutrient except vitamin C. In fact, the protein in eggs is so perfect that it is the standard against which other protein foods are measured.

If these are your favorite foods, eat them—but do so wisely.

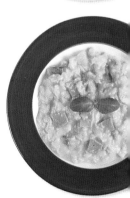

SEMI-HARD AND HARD CHEESES

● ●

HIGH IN CALCIUM, VITAMIN A, AND PROTEIN. SOME ARE HIGH IN SODIUM

*C*heddar, Swiss, Parmesan, and other hard cheeses are among the most popular—Cheddar alone accounts for 30 percent of the cheese consumed in the United States.

WHAT'S IN IT?

The nutrients vary considerably by cheese. Cheese is high in calories and fat, but it's also an excellent source of calcium and protein.

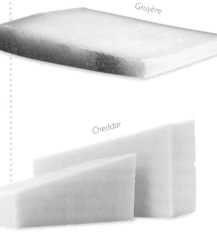

Gruyère

Cheddar

TIP

● One ounce of Cheddar, Swiss, or Monterey jack is about the size of your thumb tip, a pair of dice, or a 1-inch cube.

STYLE 1-oz	CALORIES	CHOLESTEROL mg	SODIUM mg	TOTAL FAT g
Cheddar	114	28	176	9
Swiss (Emmental)	107	26	74	7.7
Gruyère	117	31	95	9.2
Monterey jack	106	25	151	8.6
Colby	112	27	171	9.1
Parmesan, grated	129	22	527	8.5
Parmesan, grated (1 tbsp)	23	4	93	1.5
Romano	110	29	340	7.6
Low-fat Cheddar	49	6	174	2
American	93	18	337	7

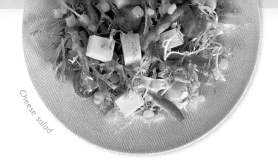

Cheese salad

WHAT'S THE BEST?

● Aged cheeses. Because they are sharper in flavor than younger, milder cheeses, you can use less of these and reap the same taste for fewer calories and less fat.

● Cheese as an alternative to dessert. Studies indicate that aged cheese such as Cheddar may help to prevent cavities.

WHAT'S NOT SO GOOD?

● Smart cooking. Low-fat cheeses are fine for snacks and sandwiches, but cook with them cautiously. They're loaded with emulsifiers that can interfere with melting.

● Large portions. Steer clear of cheese cubes at cocktail parties and big plates of nachos, where it's all too easy to eat all too much.

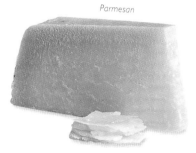

Parmesan

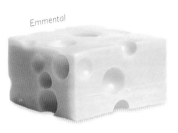

Emmental

SATURATED FAT g	PROTEIN g	CARBOHYDRATE g	FIBER g	SUGARS g	GI
6	7	0.4	0	0.2	NA
5	8	1	0	0.4	NA
5.4	8	0.1	0	0.1	NA
5.4	7	0.2	0	0.1	NA
5.7	7	0.7	0	0.1	NA
5.4	12	1.1	0	0.3	NA
1	2	0.2	0	tr	NA
4.8	9	1	0	0.2	NA
1.2	7	0.5	0	0.1	NA
4.4	6	2	0	2	NA

SOFT, SEMISOFT, AND OTHER CHEESES

●

CAN BE HIGH IN SATURATED FAT

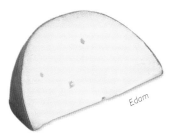

Edam

M ost of the world's cheeses, and some of the most popular, come from these categories: Provolone, Muenster, Gouda, Edam are semisoft; Brie and other cheeses with rinds are soft. Blue and brined cheese like feta are in classes by themselves.

Brie

WHAT'S IN IT?

These cheeses are higher in moisture than hard cheeses, but their fat and cholesterol contents are similar. As a general rule, they're lower in calcium and other nutrients.

TIPS

● The rind of Camembert and Brie is edible, but can be bitter. Edam and Gouda are coated with wax, which should be removed.

● The blue in blue cheese is mold from a type of penicillin. The mold is present in just the right amount to produce its characteristic flavor.

STYLE 1-oz	CALORIES	CHOLESTEROL mg	SODIUM mg	TOTAL FAT g
Blue	100	21	395	8
Brie	95	28	178	7.8
Feta	75	25	316	6
Muenster	104	27	178	6
Provolone	100	20	248	7.5
Edam	101	25	274	7.9
Gouda	101	32	232	7.8
Velveeta	85	22	420	6.2
American	93	18	337	7
Fat-free American (1 slice)	31	3	272	0.2

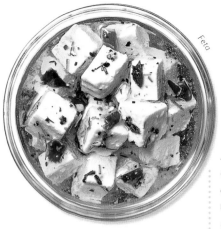

Feta

WHAT'S THE BEST?

● Strongly flavored blue and feta cheeses fall into the "little-goes-a-long-way" category. Use them in small amounts to add punch to salads. Feta is marginally lower in fat and calories than other soft and semisoft cheeses.

● Despite their rich, creamy texture, Brie and other soft cheeses are lower in fat than hard or semisoft cheese.

WHAT'S NOT SO GOOD?

● Double-crème and triple-crème cheeses. These soft cheeses can be more than 75 percent fat.

● Mold. Soft, moist cheese can spoil more readily than hard cheese, and the mold can penetrate deeper. With the exception of blue cheese, where the amount and type of mold is carefully controlled, throw away cheese with mold.

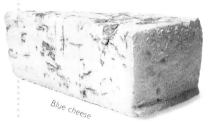

Blue cheese

SATURATED FAT g	PROTEIN g	CARBOHYDRATE g	FIBER g	SUGARS g	GI
5.3	6	0.7	0	0.1	NA
4.9	6	0.1	0	0.1	NA
4.2	4	1.2	0	1.2	NA
4.2	7	0.3	0	0.3	NA
4.8	7	0.6	0	0.2	NA
5	7	0.4	0	0.4	NA
5	7	0.6	0	0.6	NA
4	5	2.7	0	2.3	NA
4.4	6	2	0	0.2	NA
0.1	5	2.5	0	1.4	NA

FRESH CHEESES

SOME ARE VERY HIGH IN FAT

When used to describe cheese, "fresh" simply means it hasn't been aged or hasn't undergone a ripening process; it doesn't refer to quality. Fresh cheeses are more perishable than harder, aged cheeses.

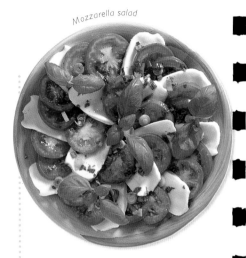

Mozzarella salad

TIP

Fresh cheeses include some of the highest in fat, but the low-fat (sometimes labeled "part skim") varieties are acceptable substitutes for their full-fat counterparts in most recipes.

WHAT'S IN IT?

The aging process removes moisture and concentrates nutrients and flavors. Fresh cheeses are often milder in flavor, and they tend to be slightly lower in calories, fat, and cholesterol. However, they're also lower in calcium and other nutrients.

STYLE 1-oz, unless noted	CALORIES	CHOLESTEROL mg	SODIUM mg	TOTAL FAT g
Ricotta (½ cup)	216	63	104	16
Part skim ricotta (½ cup)	171	38	155	9.8
Mozzarella	80	22	106	6.1
Part skim mozzarella	72	16	132	4.5
Cottage cheese (½ cup)	116	17	149	5
Cream cheese	99	31	83	10
Neufchâtel	74	22	113	6.6
Goat cheese, soft	76	13	104	6

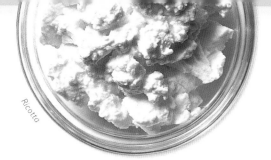
Ricotta

WHAT'S THE BEST?

● Goat cheese. If you usually reach for the very high-in-fat Boursin cheese to spread on crackers or toasted baguette, try seasoned goat cheese for a healthier alternative.

● Neufchâtel. Its flavor is virtually indistinguishable from full-fat cream cheese, and it has about one third of the calories and fat. Spread this on your bagel instead.

WHAT'S NOT SO GOOD?

● Cream cheese. Almost 90 percent of its calories are from fat; this cheese also provides very little calcium— only 23mg per oz (Parmesan, in comparison, supplies 390mg).

● Preshredded mozzarella. The high moisture content and the great amount of surface area means that packages of shredded mozzarella can spoil very quickly. If you don't plan to use all of it at once, buy a block and grate it yourself.

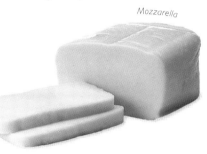
Mozzarella

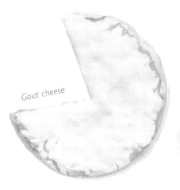
Goat cheese

SATURATED FAT g	PROTEIN g	CARBOHYDRATE g	FIBER g	SUGARS g	GI
10.2	14	3.8	0	0.3	NA
6.1	14	6.4	0	0.4	NA
3.7	6	0.6	0	0.3	NA
2.9	7	0.8	0	0.2	NA
3.2	14	3	0	0.3	NA
6.2	2	0.8	0	tr	NA
4.2	3	0.8	0	NA	NA
4.1	5	0.3	0	0.3	NA

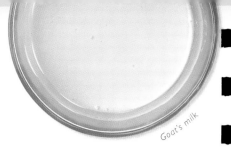
Goat's milk

MILK

● ●

CAN BE HEART-HEALTHY

You probably know that milk is an excellent source of calcium, but did you know that calcium helps to regulate heartbeat and can reduce the risk of hypertension?

WHAT'S IN IT?

Whole milk is 3.25 percent fat; reduced fat is 2 percent; low fat is 1 percent; and skim or nonfat milk is fat-free. These percentages refer to the amount of fat by weight, not the percent of calories from fat.

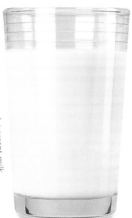
1 percent milk

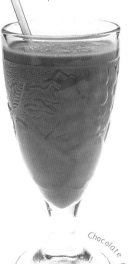
Chocolate milk

STYLE 1-cup	CALORIES	CHOLESTEROL mg	SODIUM mg	TOTAL FAT g
Whole milk	149	34	120	8.2
Fat-free (skim) milk	86	5	127	0.4
1 percent milk	102	10	124	2.6
Chocolate milk (1%)	158	8	153	3
Goat's milk	168	27	122	10

Whole milk

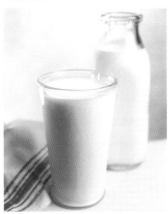

At 3.25 percent fat by weight, whole milk doesn't sound that fatty. Consider that it gets about 74 of its 149 calories from fat.

TIP

● Want the nutritional benefits of fat-free milk but hate the watery taste? Look for protein-enriched milk, which has dry milk powder added to it. It has a thicker consistency, and is slightly higher in protein and calories.

WHAT'S THE BEST?

● If you're looking to keep your calories, cholesterol, and fat as low as possible, fat-free milk is the way to go. Otherwise try 1 percent milk. It's slightly higher in calories and fat grams, but has a richer flavor.

● Chocolate and other flavored milks can tempt kids (and adults) who aren't big milk drinkers. Look for low-fat varieties.

WHAT'S NOT SO GOOD?

● Whole milk gets almost 50 percent of its calories from fat. It contains seven times the cholesterol of fat-free milk and 25 times the saturated fat.

● Goat's milk. Often touted as a healthy alternative to cow's milk, goat's milk contains just as much lactose and is rarely available in lower-fat forms.

SATURATED FAT g	PROTEIN g	CARBOHYDRATE g	FIBER g	SUGARS g	GI
5	8	11	0	11	L
0.2	8	12	0	12	L
1.6	8	12	0	12	L
1.5	8	26	0	26	L
6.5	9	10	0	10	L

MILK PRODUCTS

● ●

CAN BE HEART-HEALTHY
CONVENIENT SOURCE OF PROTEIN

Milk in cans and boxes is shelf-stable—it can be stored for six months to a year. Keep some on hand for emergencies, or for cooking.

TIP

● Dilute evaporated milk with an equal amount of water to make it drinkable; in its undiluted form, its consistency is almost identical to cream, so it makes an ideal low-fat or fat-free substitute in soups, sauces, or in coffee.

WHAT'S IN IT?

Skim and nonfat milk products are much healthier choices than their full-fat counterparts, and they are readily available.

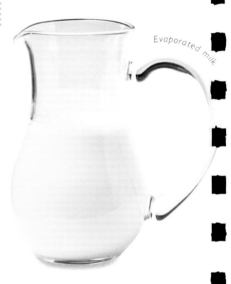

Evaporated milk

STYLE 1 cup, unless noted	CALORIES	CHOLESTEROL mg	SODIUM mg	TOTAL FAT g
Instant nonfat dry milk powder, prepared	82	4	126	0.1
Evaporated nonfat milk	200	10	294	0.5
Sweetened condensed milk (2 tbsp)	122	13	49	3.3
Sweetened condensed fat-free milk (2 tbsp)	110	4	40	0
Buttermilk	98	9.8	257	2.0

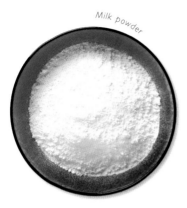

Milk powder

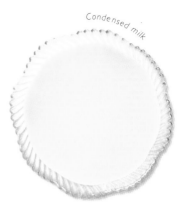

Condensed milk

Powdered milk is convenient if you've run out of fresh milk and can be stored for around six months, but many don't like the taste.

A milk product that's best avoided—condensed milk is high in sugar and low in protein. Use sparingly, if at all.

WHAT'S THE BEST?

● Despite its name, buttermilk is actually low in fat and cholesterol—it's made by adding specific bacteria to low-fat milk, which gives it a thick texture and slightly sour flavor.

● Boxed milk in aseptic packaging is shelf-stable for six months. It doesn't have the metallic flavors canned milk might, but some people notice a "cooked" taste.

WHAT'S NOT SO GOOD?

● Sweetened condensed milk. A mixture of whole milk and sugars (in almost equal amounts) is heated until more than half of the water evaporates. The result is a very thick, very sweet liquid. Because of its high sugar content, even fat-free condensed milk is very high in calories.

SATURATED FAT g	PROTEIN g	CARBOHYDRATE g	FIBER g	SUGARS g	GI
0.1	8	12	0	12	L
0.3	19	29	0	29	L
2	3	21	0	21	M
0	3	24	0	24	M
1.3	8	12	0	12	L

CREAM

HIGH IN CALORIES; CAN BE HIGH
IN FAT AND CHOLESTEROL
PROVIDES INSIGNIFICANT AMOUNTS
OF MOST NUTRIENTS

C *ream is labeled according
to the amount of milkfat
it contains, from 10 or 12 percent
(half-and-half) to as much as
40 percent (heavy cream).*

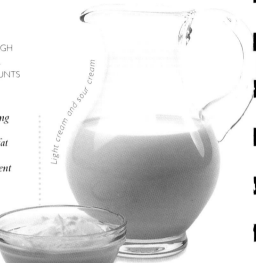

Light cream and sour cream

TIP

● One tablespoon of liquid
whipping cream will yield
2 tablespoons of whipped cream.
To add flavor without sugar, add
a little vanilla before whipping.

WHAT'S IN IT?

Most of the fat in cream is saturated.
Even half-and-half gets more than
three fourths of its calories from fat.
Think you're getting calcium with the
cream in coffee? A tablespoon of half-
and-half provides a mere 16mg—
about 1.6 percent of your daily need.

STYLE 1 tablespoon	CALORIES	CHOLESTEROL mg	SODIUM mg	TOTAL FAT g
Half-and-half	20	6	6	1.7
Nonfat half-and-half	9	1	22	0.2
Light cream	29	10	6	2.9
Whipping cream	44	17	5	4.6
Heavy cream	52	21	6	5.5
Canned whipped cream	8	2	4	0.6
Sour cream	26	5	6	2.5
Reduced-fat sour cream	20	6	6	1.8

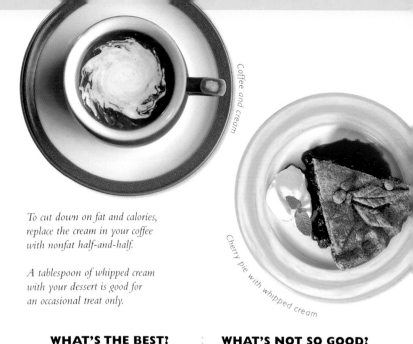

Coffee and cream

To cut down on fat and calories,
replace the cream in your coffee
with nonfat half-and-half.

A tablespoon of whipped cream
with your dessert is good for
an occasional treat only.

Cherry pie with whipped cream

WHAT'S THE BEST?

● Nonfat half-and-half. If you drink a
lot of coffee with cream, look for this
in dairy cases. Made of fat-free milk
and thickeners, it has half the calories
and none of the fat—but it does have
significantly more sodium.

● Light sour cream, made with
half-and-half rather than cream, has
40 percent less fat than does regular
sour cream. It's an excellent choice
for dips or toppings.

WHAT'S NOT SO GOOD?

● Big portions. A tablespoon
(the amount in a individual-serving
container) of half-and-half in your
coffee can become part of a balanced
diet; a serving of soup made with a
cup of cream should be reserved
for the most special occasions.

● Light and fat-free sour creams in
recipes. Fat acts to stabilize cream,
and these lower-fat varieties can
curdle over heat.

SATURATED FAT g	PROTEIN g	CARBOHYDRATE g	FIBER g	SUGARS g	GI
1	0.4	0.6	0	tr	NA
0.1	0.4	1.4	0	0.8	NA
1.8	0.4	0.6	0	tr	NA
2.9	0.3	0.4	0	tr	NA
3.4	0.3	0.4	0	tr	NA
0.4	0.9	0.4	0	tr	NA
1.6	0.4	0.5	0	tr	NA
1.1	0.4	0.6	0	tr	NA

YOGURT

● ●

RICH IN CALCIUM, RIBOFLAVIN,
AND VITAMIN B12

Yogurt is made by introducing beneficial bacteria to milk. The bacteria eat the lactose, or milk sugar, making yogurt a good choice for those who are lactose-intolerant.

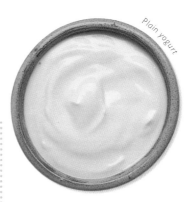

Plain yogurt

High in vitamins and minerals, and low in fat— plain yogurt is a healthful alternative to sour cream.

TIPS

● Yogurt is a healthful alternative to sour cream and mayonnaise in dips and salad dressings. Even full-fat yogurt has a fraction of the calories, fat, and cholesterol of sour cream or mayonnaise.

● Yogurt cheese, made by draining off the whey, can be used as a substitute for mayonnaise or cream cheese.

WHAT'S IN IT?

Plain yogurt is an excellent source of protein, vitamins, and minerals and can be low in fat. It's also very high in calcium, riboflavin, and vitamin B12, and read labels—some brands of plain yogurt even supply fiber. Steer clear of flavored yogurts, which can be surprisingly high in sugar.

STYLE 8-oz container	CALORIES	CHOLESTEROL mg	SODIUM mg	TOTAL FAT g
Low-fat with fruit	232	9	132	2.4
Fat-free, sugar-free w/fruit	125	11	102	0.4
Plain fat-free	127	4.5	175	0.4
Plain low-fat	143	14	159	3.5
Plain whole milk	138	30	104	7.3

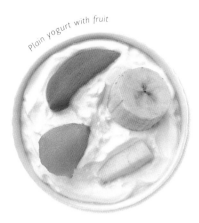

Plain yogurt with fruit

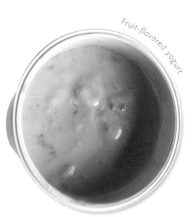

Fruit-flavored yogurt

Why buy fruit yogurts with added sugar? It's more healthful to chop up fresh fruit and add it to plain yogurt.

Fruit-flavored yogurt often contains surprisingly high amounts of sugar—hardly a healthful food!

WHAT'S THE BEST?

● Live cultures. Labels that say "contains live cultures" or "contains active cultures" indicate a yogurt with beneficial bacteria that can help regulate the bacteria in the digestive tract.

● Plain low-fat or nonfat yogurt. One cup contains more than 400mg calcium—40 percent of the daily requirement for most adults.

WHAT'S NOT SO GOOD?

● Sweetened yogurt. Some fruit flavors have more than 2 tablespoons of sugar per cup; vanilla, coffee, and lemon flavors have a little over a tablespoon.

● Fruit yogurts. Because the fruit takes up space in the 8-oz cup, you get less calcium and B vitamins. Better to add fruit to a cup of plain yogurt.

SATURATED FAT g	PROTEIN g	CARBOHYDRATE g	FIBER g	SUGARS g	GI
1.6	10	43	0	43	L
0.2	8	22	0	17	L
0.3	13	17	0	17	L
2.3	12	16	0	16	L
4.8	8	11	0	11	L

EGGS

● ●

GOOD SOURCE OF PROTEIN.
YOLKS ARE HIGH IN CHOLESTEROL

*E*ggs are high in protein, zinc, B vitamins, and other nutrients—in fact, the only nutrient missing from eggs is vitamin C. However, just one supplies more than one third of the recommended daily allowance of cholesterol.

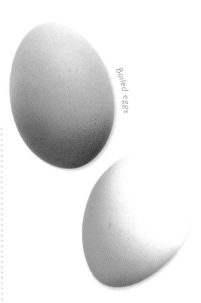

Boiled eggs

TIP

 Recent research shows that most people are less affected by the amount of cholesterol in foods than by the amount of saturated fat. The American Heart Association now advises limiting eggs only to stay under the 300mg cholesterol per day recommendation.

WHAT'S IN IT?

The egg yolk contains all the fat, fat-soluble vitamins, cholesterol, and virtually all of the carbohydrate; the egg whites are all protein, water, and contain most of the egg's mineral content. Brown eggs are no different from white eggs nutritionally. It is the color of the hen's ears and feathers that determines the color of her eggs.

STYLE 1 large egg	CALORIES	CHOLESTEROL mg	SODIUM mg	TOTAL FAT g
Boiled egg	78	212	62	5.3
Poached egg	75	212	140	5
Scrambled egg	101	215	170	7.4
Omelet	93	217	98	7.3
Fried egg	92	211	162	7
Egg white	17	0	54	0
Liquid egg substitute (¼ cup)	54	0.6	113	2.1

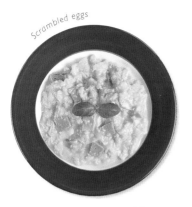

Scrambled eggs

Just a small amount of fat is needed to scramble eggs, so they make a nutritionally sound meal.

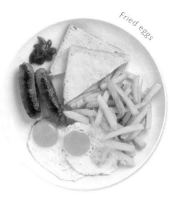

Fried eggs

Serve sausages, fries, and bread alongside fried eggs and you'll be overloaded with cholesterol and saturated fats.

WHAT'S THE BEST?

● Smart cooking. Boil or poach eggs; use a nonstick pan so you can scramble or fry with a minute amount of fat.

● "Enhanced" eggs. Hens fed a special diet lay eggs that are lower in cholesterol and higher in heart-healthy omega-3 fatty acids.

● Egg substitutes are fat-free and cholesterol-free alternatives to whole eggs, made primarily of egg whites.

WHAT'S NOT SO GOOD?

● Fried eggs. Eggs aren't horrible by themselves, but cook them in butter and serve them with buttered toast and you've got unhealthy amounts of fat on your plate.

● Bad combinations. Avoid serving eggs with bacon, steak, or sausage. Instead, make an omelet with a spinach and tomato filling and serve it with whole-grain toast.

SATURATED FAT g	PROTEIN g	CARBOHYDRATE g	FIBER g	SUGARS g	GI
1.6	6	0.6	0	0.6	NA
1.5	6	0.6	0	0.4	NA
2.2	7	1.3	0	1	NA
2	6	0.4	0	0.4	NA
1.9	6	0.6	0	0.4	NA
0	3.4	0.3	0	0.2	NA
0.4	8	0.4	0	0.4	NA

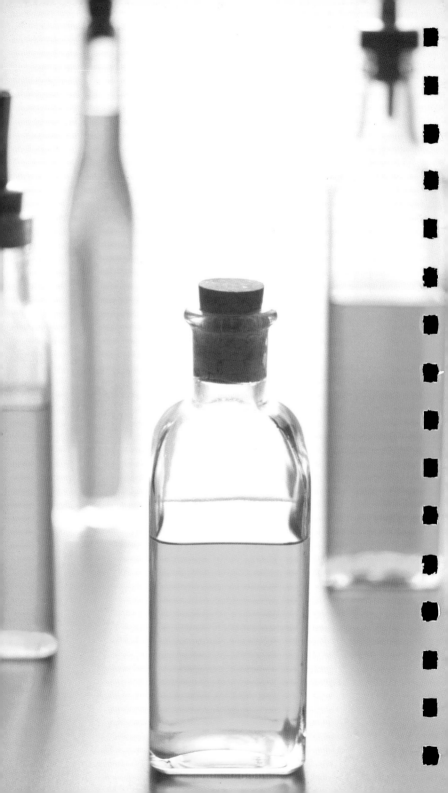

FATS AND OILS

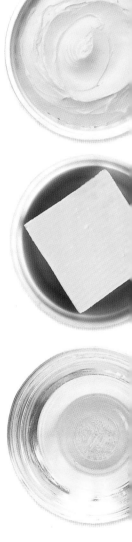

Fat isn't the villain some make it out to be—in fact, it's a vital nutrient—but sorting out good fats and bad fats can be challenging.

Be especially careful about eliminating fat if you are trying to lose weight. Fat is far more satisfying than carbohydrates, so it makes you feel full longer and can help you eat less.

Most fats fall into three groups. Monounsaturated and polyunsaturated fats are liquid at room temperature, and saturated fats are solid at room temperature. Virtually all dietary fats—butter, lard, and vegetable oils—are a combination of the three types.

A fourth type of fat, trans fat, is made by processing liquid vegetable oils with hydrogen. These partially hydrogenated oils are by far the most harmful. Unlike the other three types, trans fats raise levels of LDL ("bad") cholesterol and lower levels of HDL ("good") cholesterol.

BUTTER

●

HIGH IN CHOLESTEROL
AND SATURATED FAT. GOOD
SOURCE OF VITAMIN A

Butter has been reviled by nutritionists for its high cholesterol and saturated fat content, but its flavor is unmatched by margarine and other imitators.

Salted butter

TIP

● The milk solids in butter burn easily, so butter is said to have a low smoke point. When your recipe calls for foods to be sautéed in butter, use a mixture of half butter, half vegetable oil to raise the smoke point and lessen the likelihood of burning.

WHAT'S IN IT?

Butter is usually 80–82 percent fat and 18–20 percent milk solids. Although we think of butter as a saturated fat, it's really only about 66 percent saturated. The remainder is 30 percent monounsaturated and 4 percent polyunsaturated.

STYLE 1 tablespoon	CALORIES	CHOLESTEROL mg	SODIUM mg	TOTAL FAT g
Unsalted	102	31	2	11.5
Salted	102	31	117	11.5
Whipped	67	21	78	7.6

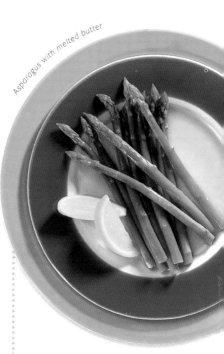

Asparagus with melted butter

WHAT'S THE BEST?

● Unsalted butter tends to be fresher than salted butter; salt acts as a preservative, so salted butter may have been on supermarket shelves longer.

● Whipped butter has air mixed into it, so it has fewer calories and other nutrients than solid butter. Don't use it for baking, though, unless the recipe specifically calls for it.

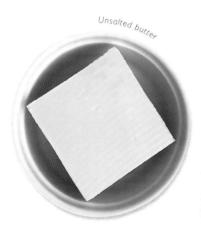

Unsalted butter

Asparagus drizzled with melted butter is delicious, but high in fat—use any butter sauces sparingly.

WHAT'S NOT SO GOOD?

● Large amounts. If you have buttered toast with breakfast, buttered vegetables at lunch, and a buttered baked potato with dinner, you're overdoing it.

● Butter sauces. Reserve these for the occasional meal. Use broth or oil-based sauces regularly.

SATURATED FAT g	PROTEIN g	CARBOHYDRATE g	FIBER g	SUGARS g	GI
7.2	tr	tr	0	0	0
7.2	tr	tr	0	0	0
4.8	tr	tr	0	0	0

MARGARINE AND SHORTENING

●

CAN BE HEART-HEALTHY

Don't be impressed by margarine labels claiming to be "cholesterol-free"—cholesterol is found in animal products only, and margarine is made from vegetable oils. Instead, look for "no trans fats" or "trans fat-free."

WHAT'S IN IT?

Margarines run the gamut from fat-free to getting 80 percent of their calories from fat (the same as butter). Margarines are generally low in saturated fats and are cholesterol-free. As with other fats, margarines contain a mixture of saturated, monounsaturated, and polyunsaturated fats. Some include high levels of trans fats.

TIPS

● Shortening is pure hydrogenated vegetable oil—in short, trans fat. It is used primarily for baking and deep-frying. Use it in moderation, but it's best to avoid it altogether.

● Look for margarine blended with yogurt for a healthful spread with dairy flavor. Margarine-butter blends are made with hydrogenated oils and should be avoided.

STYLE 1 tablespoon	CALORIES	CHOLESTEROL mg	SODIUM mg	TOTAL FAT g
Regular (80% fat)	98.7	0	91.5	11
Spread (40% fat)	50	0	138	5.6
Soft, safflower (1 tsp)	34	0	51	3.8
Fat-free, bottle	7	tr	128	0.4
Fat-free, spread	6	0	85	0.4
Margarine-butter blend	102	13	127	11.5
Margarine-yogurt blend	45	0	90	5
Shortening	113	0	0	12.8

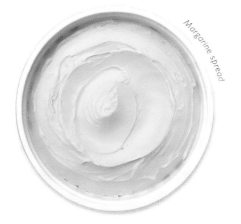

Margarine spread

WHAT'S THE BEST?

● Trans fat-free. Look for these words on the label, or read the list of ingredients and avoid any margarines that list "hydrogenated" or "partially hydrogenated" oils.

● Cholesterol-lowering margarines. These rather pricey products contain phytosterols, plant chemicals that block the absorption of cholesterol in the intestines. Use them instead of, and not in addition to, other fats in your diet.

WHAT'S NOT SO GOOD?

● Saturated fat. Margarine should contain about twice as much polyunsaturated fat as saturated fat. If polyunsaturated fat isn't listed on the Nutrition Facts label, find a different brand.

● Shortening. This solid vegetable fat is high in trans fats. You're better off using canola oil to fry foods, and butter or an oil with a neutral flavor in baked goods

SATURATED FAT g	PROTEIN g	CARBOHYDRATE g	FIBER g	SUGARS g	GI
2	tr	tr	0	0	0
0.9	tr	tr	0	0	0
0.4	tr	tr	0	0	0
tr	0	0.8	0	0	0
0.3	tr	0.6	0	0	0
4	tr	tr	0	0	0
I	0	0	0	0	0
2	0	0	0	0	0

VEGETABLE OILS

● ●

CAN BE HEART-HEALTHY
SOME ARE HIGH IN VITAMIN E
AND OMEGA-3 FATS

Unlike animal fats that contain trace amounts of protein and carbohydrate, vegetable oils are 100 percent fat. They all contain saturated fat, monounsaturated fat, and polyunsaturated fat, but the breakdown varies widely by oil. Canola oil, for example, is 6 percent saturated, 62 percent monounsaturated, and 31 percent polyunsaturated; safflower oil is 9 percent saturated, 12 percent monounsaturated, and 78 percent polyunsaturated.

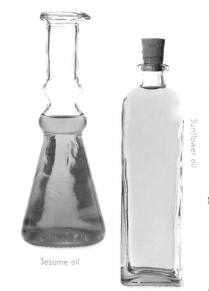

Sesame oil

Sunflower oil

WHAT'S IN IT?

Most vegetable oils supply about 120 calories per tablespoon and they are sodium- and cholesterol-free. Those vegetable oils that are high in polyunsaturated fats are higher in heart-healthy omega-3 and omega-6 fatty acids.

STYLE 1 tablespoon	CALORIES	CHOLESTEROL mg	SODIUM mg	TOTAL FAT g
Soybean oil	104	0	0	13.6
Canola oil	124	0	0	14
Sunflower oil	120	0	0	13.6
Safflower oil	120	0	0	13.6
Corn oil	120	0	0	13.6
Peanut oil	120	0	0	13.5
Sesame oil	120	0	0	13.6
Palm oil	120	0	0	13.6

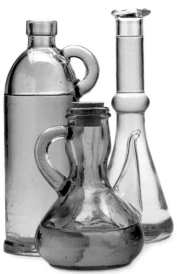

Various vegetable oils

Choose oils wisely—some are rich in vitamin E and omega-3 fatty acids, others provide mainly saturated fats.

WHAT'S THE BEST?

● Canola oil. Highest in omega-3s, this mildly-flavored all-purpose oil also has a high smoke point, so it can be heated to higher temperatures than most oils before it breaks down.

● Cold pressed or expeller pressed oils. These oils are made without heat; they have better flavor and more nutrients.

TIP

● Never reuse oil for frying. When heated, oils can decompose, breaking down into harmful compounds called nitrosamines. Used oils become rancid and develop off flavors.

WHAT'S NOT SO GOOD?

● Palm oil. Used almost exclusively in packaged foods and baked goods, this oil is highly saturated.

● Big portions. Always measure oil for sautéing rather than pouring it into a pan—it's easy to underestimate the amount you're actually using.

SATURATED FAT g	PROTEIN g	CARBOHYDRATE g	FIBER g	SUGARS g	GI
2	0	0	0	0	0
1	0	0	0	0	0
1.4	0	0	0	0	0
0.8	0	0	0	0	0
1.7	0	0	0	0	0
2.3	0	0	0	0	0
1.9	0	0	0	0	0
6.7	0	0	0	0	0

OLIVE OIL

● ● ●

HEART-HEALTHY
GOOD SOURCE OF VITAMIN E

*O*live oil, made by pressing the oil out of olives, can vary in color, flavor, and acidity, but the different varieties are the same nutritionally.

WHAT'S IN IT?

Olive oil is about 14 percent saturated, 77 percent monounsaturated, and 9 percent polyunsaturated. One tablespoon provides about about 10 percent of the vitamin E requirement for the day.

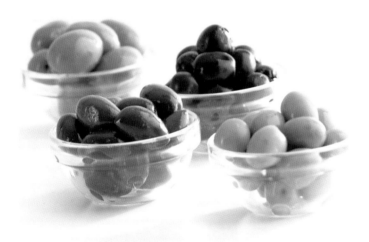

Rich in vitamin E and flavorsome, olives and olive oils are a good source of monounsaturated fats.

STYLE 1 tablespoon	CALORIES	CHOLESTEROL mg	SODIUM mg	TOTAL FAT g
Olive oil	119	0	0	13.5

WHAT'S THE BEST?

● Variety. An extra-virgin olive oil that's cold pressed will taste wonderful, but its depth of flavor will be muted if you use it to sauté. Reserve it for dipping bread or drizzling over vegetables and use a virgin or pure oil for cooking.

● Dark bottles. Like all fats, olive oil can go rancid quickly. Protect it by keeping it in a dark glass bottle or metal container, or out of direct sunlight.

WHAT'S NOT SO GOOD?

● Light olive oil. Don't be duped into thinking this otherwise perfectly fine oil is lower in calories or fat content. Unlike other foods, where "light" means one third fewer calories or 50 percent less fat, light olive oil has simply undergone additional processing to give it a milder flavor and lighter color.

● Frying. Olive oil has a low smoke point, so it begins to break down at a fairly low temperature. But the filtration that removes flavor from light olive oil also gives it a higher smoke point. If you need an olive oil that can withstand high temperatures, choose light.

TIP

● Look for "cold-pressed" on the label. This means that no heat was used to extract the oil, so the oil will have a truer olive flavor.

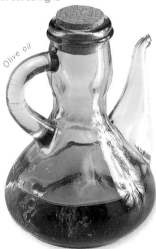
Olive oil

SATURATED FAT g	PROTEIN g	CARBOHYDRATE g	FIBER g	SUGARS g	GI
1.8	0	0	0	0	0

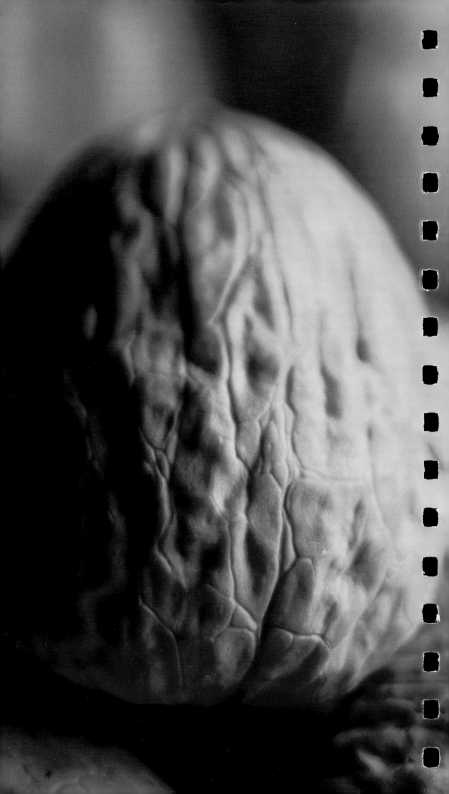

NUTS, SEEDS, AND LEGUMES

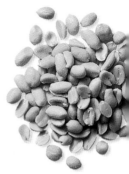

Proof that good things come in small packages, nuts, seeds, and dried beans are high in many beneficial nutrients and low in potentially harmful ones.

Nuts and seeds have been demonized in the past because of their high fat content, but recent research shows that their fats are beneficial—and that nuts are packed with many other nutrients.

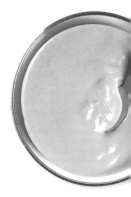

Legumes and pulses, the dried seeds of beans and other plants, are also high in vitamins and minerals, particularly calcium and folate. Deficiencies of this B vitamin have been linked to birth defects like spina bifida, and to increased risk for heart disease and some types of cancer.

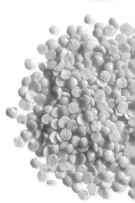

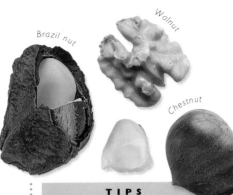

Brazil nut

Walnut

Chestnut

NUTS

● ● ●

HEART-HEALTHY
CONCENTRATED SOURCE
OF MANY NUTRIENTS

For years, nutrition experts counseled avoiding nuts because of their high calorie and fat content, but studies show that eating nuts five times a week can cut the risk of heart attack in half.

WHAT'S IN IT?

One ounce of nuts—or roughly 1/4 cup—contains around 175 calories and as many as 21g of fat. Almonds are high in vitamin E, calcium, and protein; walnuts in cardio-protective omega-3s; and cashews in iron and folate. Most nuts are also high in fiber.

TIPS

● Dry-roasted and oil-roasted nuts have similar calories and fat, but dry-roasted nuts often include high-sodium seasonings as well as sweeteners and preservatives. Better to buy raw nuts and toast them in a skillet over medium-low heat, shaking the pan constantly.

● Botanically, peanuts are legumes, but because they are eaten like nuts more often than like dried beans, they are included here.

STYLE 1-oz raw nuts	CALORIES	CHOLESTEROL mg	SODIUM mg	TOTAL FAT g
Almonds	164	0	tr	14.4
Brazil nuts	186	0	1	18.7
Cashews	160	0	3	13.3
Hazelnuts	178	0	0	17.2
Pecans	196	0	0	20.4
Peanuts	161	0	5	14
Walnuts	185	0	1	18.5
Peanut butter (2 tbsp)	190	0	150	16.3
Chestnuts, roasted	69	0	1	0.6
Macadamias	203	0	1	21.5
Pistachios	158	0	tr	12.6

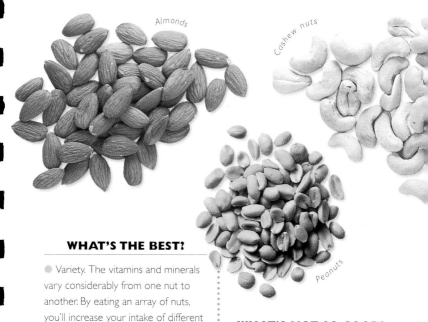

Almonds

Cashew nuts

Peanuts

WHAT'S THE BEST?

● Variety. The vitamins and minerals vary considerably from one nut to another. By eating an array of nuts, you'll increase your intake of different vitamins and minerals.

● Small packages. Because of their high fat content, nuts can go rancid quickly. Unless you know you'll use up the family-size jar within a few months, buy a smaller container. Keep nuts in the freezer for up to six months; bring them to room temperature before using.

WHAT'S NOT SO GOOD?

● Big portions. Yes, nuts have their place in a healthful diet, but it's a small one. One ounce a day, about 1/4 cup, is enough to reap their benefits.

● Processed nuts. Whether salted cashews or sweetened commercial peanut butter, the more that's done to nuts, the less healthful they are.

SATURATED FAT g	PROTEIN g	CARBOHYDRATE g	FIBER g	SUGARS g	GI
1.1	6	6	3.3	1.4	NA
5.6	4	4	1.5	0	NA
2.3	4	8	0.9	1.7	L
1.3	4	5	2.7	1.3	NA
1.8	3	4	2.7	1.1	NA
1.9	7	5	2.4	0	L
1.7	4	4	1.9	0.7	NA
3.3	8	6	1.9	2.5	NA
0.1	1	15	1.4	3	NA
3.4	2	4	2.4	1.3	NA
1.5	6	8	2.9	2.2	NA

COCONUTS

HIGH IN SATURATED FAT.
GOOD SOURCE OF FIBER

At first glance, coconuts' high saturated fat content would seem to make them a forbidden food. But they are also high in phytosterols, compounds that have been shown to reduce levels of blood cholesterol.

WHAT'S IN IT?

One piece of fresh coconut meat provides generous amounts of fiber and vitamin E.

TIPS

● Cracking coconuts is a labor-intensive undertaking, as is making coconut milk. Look for frozen coconut meat, or unsweetened cans of coconut milk.

● Beware the difference between coconut cream and cream of coconut. Coconut cream has a butter-like texture; it rises to the top of coconut milk. Cream of coconut is a highly sweetened canned product used in tropical drinks.

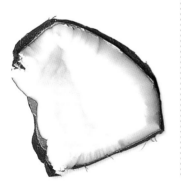

STYLE 1-oz, unless noted	CALORIES	CHOLESTEROL mg	SODIUM mg	TOTAL FAT g
Coconut meat (2 x 2 x ½ inches)	159	0	9	15.1
Coconut milk (½ cup)	223	0	15	24.1
Cream of coconut	110	0	15	5
Sweetened, dried	134	0	73	9.1
Unsweetened dried	187	0	11	18.3
Coconut oil (1 tbsp)	117	0	0	13.6
Coconut cream (1 tbsp)	36	0	10	3.4

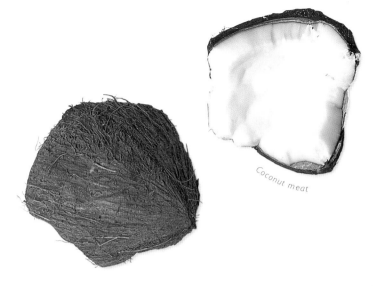

Coconut meat

Dried coconut

WHAT'S THE BEST?

● Coconut milk. Add it to sauces, or use it (dilute with water) to make Thai-style rice.

● Toasted fresh coconut. If you've gone to the trouble to crack open a coconut, use a vegetable peeler to cut off thin strips of the flesh. Arrange them on a baking sheet and toast at 300°F for 10–15 minutes, stirring often. Season lightly with salt and serve warm.

WHAT'S NOT SO GOOD?

● Sweetened dried coconut. Coconut is naturally sweet, but the stuff that you'll find in supermarkets is laden with added sugar. Seek out unsweetened coconut in a natural foods store.

SATURATED FAT g	PROTEIN g	CARBOHYDRATE g	FIBER g	SUGARS g	GI
13.4	2	7	4.1	2.8	NA
21.4	2	3	0	NA	NA
4.0	0	17	0	17	NA
8.1	1	14	1.2	12.3	NA
16.2	2	7	4.6	2.1	NA
11.8	0	0	0	0	NA
3.0	0.5	1.6	0.4	1.2	NA

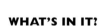

Pumpkin seeds

SEEDS

● ● ●

HEART-HEALTHY. HIGH IN FIBER,
VITAMINS, AND MINERALS

I f you grab a handful of seeds rather than a handful of chips for your next snack, you'll get a healthy dose of vital nutrients rather than empty calories.

Sunflower seeds

WHAT'S IN IT?

One ounce of dry-roasted sunflower seeds (without salt) provides hefty amounts of vitamin E, the mineral selenium, and folate, as well as protein and fiber. Choose the salted variety and the sodium content of your nibble vaults from 1mg up to a whopping 221mg.

STYLE 1-oz, unless noted	CALORIES	CHOLESTEROL mg	SODIUM mg	TOTAL FAT g
Sunflower seeds, dry roasted w/o salt	165	0	1	14.1
Sesame seeds (1 tbsp)	97	0	1	4.5
Flaxseeds (1 tbsp)	59	0	4	4
Pumpkin seeds, roasted w/o salt	148	0	5	11.9
Tahini (1 tbsp)	89	0	17	8

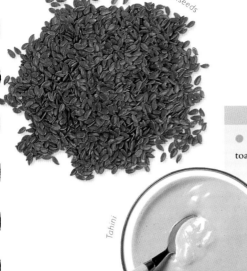

Flaxseeds

Tahini

TIP

● Boost seeds' flavor by toasting them. Put them in a skillet set over medium heat. Cook, shaking the pan constantly (they can burn easily) until they are golden brown and aromatic.

WHAT'S THE BEST?

● Flaxseeds are rich in a type of fat that the body converts to omega-3 fatty acids. These essential fatty acids make the blood less likely to clot and can reduce the risk of heart attacks. Flaxseeds also contain compounds that are being studied for their potential in reducing tumors.

WHAT'S NOT SO GOOD?

● Whole seeds. These pass through the body undigested, taking their nutritional benefits with them. Chewing seeds will release some of the nutrients, but use ground flax meal or tahini, a paste made from sesame seeds, in order to obtain the most nutrients.

SATURATED FAT g	PROTEIN g	CARBOHYDRATE g	FIBER g	SUGARS g	GI
1.5	5	7	3.1	0.8	NA
0.6	2	2	1	tr	NA
0.4	2	4	3.3	0.1	NA
2.3	9	4	1.1	0.3	NA
1.1	3	3	1.4	tr	NA

SOYBEANS

● ● ●

CAN HELP LOWER CHOLESTEROL

*S*oy protein is the only complete *vegetable protein—it contains* all the essential amino acids. Soy also supplies iron, calcium, magnesium, vitamin E, riboflavin, thiamin, folate, and beneficial fats.

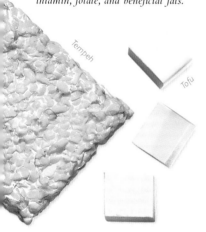

Tempeh

Tofu

WHAT'S IN IT?

If firm tofu has been prepared with calcium, it can have as much as 200mg per ½-cup serving; soft tofu can have almost 140mg.

TIPS

● Do you drink soymilk? It may not be as healthful as you think. Flavored soymilks are often sweetened with rice- or barley-based syrups.

● Soy contains isoflavones, antioxidant compounds that can help prevent some cancers, osteoporosis, and heart disease. Research indicates that 25g soy protein contains beneficial amounts of isoflavones.

STYLE ½ cup, unless noted	CALORIES	CHOLESTEROL mg	SODIUM mg	TOTAL FAT g
Tofu, firm	97	0	10	5.6
Tofu, soft	76	0	10	4.6
Tofu, silken firm (3 oz)	52	0	30	2.3
Tempeh	160	0	7	9
Soymilk, vanilla (1 cup)	150	0	85	3
Edamame	127	0	13	5.8
Soy cheese (1 oz)	70	0	194	3.4
TVP crumbles	116	0	238	6.5
Vegetable burger (1)	91	0	383	0.5

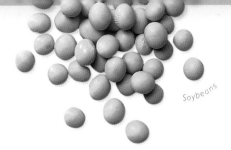

Soybeans

WHAT'S THE BEST?

● Edamame. Boiled and seasoned fresh soybeans are a delicious nibble and an easy way to incorporate soy protein into your diet.

● Meat analogs. If you haven't had a veggie burger or Textured Vegetable Protein (TVP) crumbles lately, you'll be amazed at the improved flavor and texture when you do.

WHAT'S NOT SO GOOD?

● Soybean oil and soy sauce don't provide soy protein, nor do they have any of soy's nutritional benefits.

● Soy flour. It's higher in protein and lower in carbohydrate than wheat flour, but don't bake with it unless the recipe calls for it. Soy flour lacks gluten, a protein necessary for structure in yeast breads.

It may help prevent cancer, osteoporosis, and heart disease— not bad for a humble veggie burger!

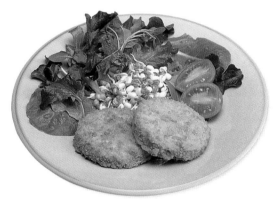

SATURATED FAT g	PROTEIN g	CARBOHYDRATE g	FIBER g	SUGARS g	GI
0.8	10	4	0.5	0.8	NA
0.6	8	2	0.2	0.9	NA
0.3	6	2	tr	1.1	NA
1.8	15	8	NA	NA	NA
0	7	24	3.3	15	L
0.6	11	10	3.8	NA	NA
1	3	7	0	NA	NA
1.6	11	3	2.5	0.6	NA
0.1	14	7.5	4.3	0.48	NA

LEGUMES AND PULSES

● ● ●

CAN BE HEART-HEALTHY
EXCELLENT LOW-FAT SOURCE
OF PROTEIN

*C*onvenient, inexpensive,
*flavorful, versatile, and
nutritious, dried beans are a
staple in many cuisines.*

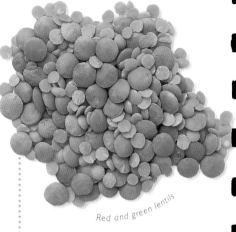

Red and green lentils

Yellow lentils

WHAT'S IN IT?

All beans are rich in fiber, protein, and complex carbohydrates. Most are high in folate, which can help prevent birth defects like cleft palate and spina bifida, as well as protect against heart disease and some forms of cancer. Some beans are high in calcium, too. Peas and lima beans are high in vitamin A.

Lentils are an excellent source of protein—use them to make vegetable burgers or a delicious winter soup.

STYLE 1 cup	CALORIES	CHOLESTEROL mg	SODIUM mg	TOTAL FAT g
Lentils	230	0	4	0.7
Split peas	231	0	4	0.8
Black beans	227	0	2	0.9
Chickpeas	269	0	11	4.2
Kidney beans	225	0	4	0.9
Navy beans	258	0	2	1

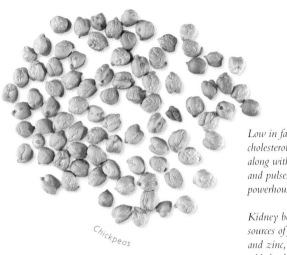

Chickpeas

Low in fat and with zero cholesterol, chickpeas— along with other legumes and pulses—are nutritional powerhouses.

Kidney beans are great sources of fiber, potassium, and zinc, but watch out for added salt if they're canned.

TIP

● Canned beans are far more convenient than the soaked and boiled variety, but they tend to be very high in sodium. To remove up to 40 percent of this mineral, pour the beans and their liquid into a colander and rinse them thoroughly, then shake off the extra moisture before using them in a recipe.

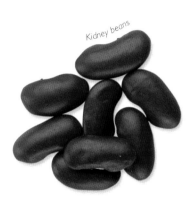

Kidney beans

SATURATED FAT g	PROTEIN g	CARBOHYDRATE g	FIBER g	SUGARS g	GI
0.1	18	40	16	3.6	L
0.1	16	41	16	5.7	L
0.2	15	41	15	NA	L
0.4	15	45	12	8	L
0.1	15	41	13	0.5	L
0.3	15	48	12	NA	L

LEGUMES AND PULSES

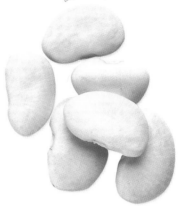

Lima beans

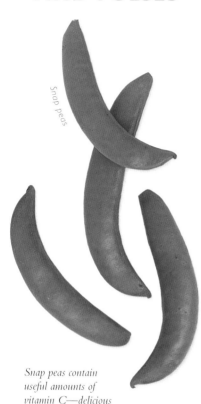

Snap peas

Lima beans contain fiber, potassium, and iron—use them in salads and stews.

TIPS

● Don't turn up your nose at frozen peas. Often processed within hours of harvest, they have wonderful flavor and texture.

● Traditionally made with chickpeas, hummus is very easy—and economical—to make.

Snap peas contain useful amounts of vitamin C—delicious eaten raw in salads.

STYLE 1 cup	CALORIES	CHOLESTEROL mg	SODIUM mg	TOTAL FAT g
Pinto beans	252	0	3	0.9
Pink beans	234	0	3	0.9
Lima beans	209	0	29	0.5
Cowpeas	160	0	7	0.6
Green peas	134	0	5	0.3
Snap peas	67	0	6	0.4
Hummus (¼ cup)	93	0	212	5.4

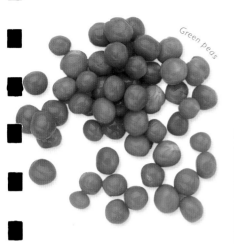

Green peas

WHAT'S THE BEST?

● Fiber. All legumes are rich in both types of fiber, soluble (which lowers LDL, or "bad," cholesterol) and insoluble (which prevents constipation).

● Small portions. One cup of dried beans supplies as much as 16g of fiber (20g–35g is the recommended amount per day; most people consume significantly less than that). If you're not accustomed to eating so many beans, you'll have less discomfort if you start with 1/4-cup or 1/2-cup servings.

WHAT'S NOT SO GOOD?

● Baked beans. Doused with molasses and spiked with bacon, baked beans are higher in sugar and fat than most other beans.

● Oligosaccharides. An unfamiliar word for a common problem, these complex sugars are indigestible, and as they pass through the digestive system they produce gas. To lessen them, soak beans before cooking and discard the soaking liquid.

You can't beat a hearty meal of baked beans, but beware of the sugar content in many canned varieties—check the label and opt for low-sugar versions.

SATURATED FAT g	PROTEIN g	CARBOHYDRATE g	FIBER g	SUGARS g	GI
0.2	16	42	9	0.6	L
0.2	15	48	15	0.6	L
0.1	12	40	9	2.8	L
0.2	5	34	8.3	5.3	L
tr	9	25	9	9.5	L
tr	5	11	4	6.4	L
0.8	4	8	3.2	NA	L

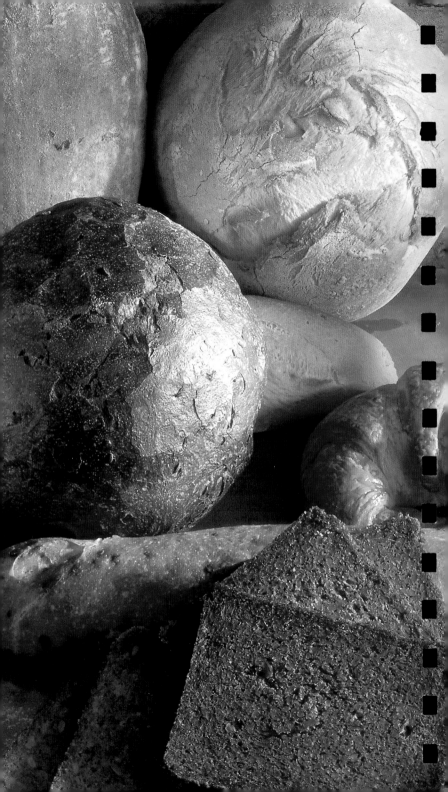

STARCHY FOODS

The staff of life, the base of the Food Guide Pyramid, or a dietary disaster? The truth is that high-carbohydrate foods can be all three.

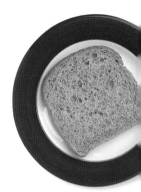

The Food Guide Pyramid recommends 6–11 servings from this group every day. Sound like a lot? Consider that the Pyramid calls a serving of rice or pasta $\frac{1}{2}$ cup, but the amount on your dinner plate is rarely less than 1 cup—and the typical restaurant serving of pasta is closer to 4 cups! Or consider that a serving is a 1-ounce slice of bread, but that a bagel from a bakery can easily weigh 6 ounces.

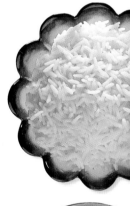

The Pyramid doesn't differentiate between a bowl of sugary cereal and a bowl of oatmeal, or a slice of spongy white bread or one high in chewy whole grains. Your body, however, knows that all carbs are not created equal. Avoid foods made of refined flours and choose whole grains and whole-grain products instead.

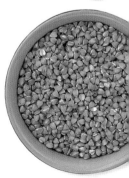

BREADS

● ●

LOW IN FAT AND CHOLESTEROL.
CAN BE LOW IN NUTRIENTS

Pumpernickel

If your goal is to make every calorie count, you'll need to choose bread very wisely and pay attention to portion sizes.

French baguette

WHAT'S IN IT?

Whole-grain breads provide some fiber, vitamin E, B vitamins, and minerals like selenium, zinc, and magnesium.

TIP

● Slices of bread typically weigh between 25g and 30g, but can weigh up to 35g. One ounce, or 28.35g, is used below as a standard. If your bread doesn't have a Nutrition Facts label, divide the number of slices by the weight of the loaf to determine how much each slice weighs.

STYLE 1-oz	CALORIES	CHOLESTEROL mg	SODIUM mg	TOTAL FAT g
White	76	.2	153	1
Whole-wheat	70	0	149	1.2
Rye	73	0	187	0.9
Pumpernickel	71	0	190	0.9
Mixed grain	71	0	138	1.1
French or sourdough	78	0	173	0.9
Bagel, plain, onion, or sesame (4½-inch diam, 4–5 oz)	360	0	700	2.1
Bialy (4-inch diam, 2–3 oz)	138	0	300	0
English muffin	134	0	264	1.0
Croissant (1 medium)	231	38	424	12.0

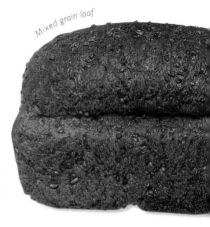

Mixed grain loaf

WHAT'S THE BEST?

● Whole grains. Mixed grain breads usually contain very small amounts of barley, oats, millet, and even rye, so be sure that they are made with whole-wheat flour.

● Portion awareness. The information below is for 1 oz of bread, or a slice about the size of a stack of 3 floppy disks. Slices of specialty bread from a bakery can often weigh 2 or 3 oz, and bagels can weigh almost a 1/2 pound!

Whole-wheat loaf

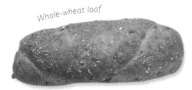

WHAT'S NOT SO GOOD?

● "Wheat bread." Don't be fooled—any bread made of wheat flour can be called wheat bread. Look for "100 percent whole-wheat."

● Ingredients lists. Their small print can be difficult to read, and with all those parentheses and brackets it can be hard to figure out where "enriched flour" ends and the next ingredient begins. Look at the Nutrition Facts label and choose high-fiber (about 2g per slice) breads.

SATURATED FAT g	PROTEIN g	CARBOHYDRATE g	FIBER g	SUGARS g	GI
0.1	2	14	0.6	1	H
0.3	3	13	2	1	M
0.2	2	14	1.6	tr	L
0.1	2	13	1.8	0.2	L
0.2	3	13	1.8	2.8	L
0.2	2	15	0.9	tr	H
0.3	14	70	3	NA	H
0	7	32	NA	NA	H
0.1	4	26	1.5	6	H
6.6	5	26	1.5	6.4	H

QUICK BREADS AND UNLEAVENED BREADS

●

CAN BE HIGH IN CARBS AND TRANS FATS. OFTEN HIGH IN SODIUM

Unlike yeast-risen breads, quick breads are leavened with baking powder or baking soda, and both are high in sodium.

TIP

● Exercise skepticism in the face of bran and "whole-grain" muffins. The odds are high that those touted as healthy contain a considerable amount of refined flour, as well as sugar and trans fats.

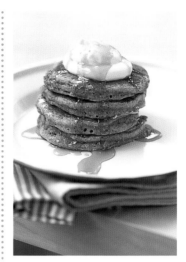

Pancakes are low in fat; it's the toppings you add that can pile on the pounds.

WHAT'S IN IT?

Though some unleavened breads are low in calories and can be high in fiber, others are high in fat and calories, and can be high in added sugar, too.

STYLE 1 medium	CALORIES	CHOLESTEROL mg	SODIUM mg	TOTAL FAT g
Bran muffin (4 oz)	305	0	444	8.3
Blueberry muffin (4 oz)	313	34	50	7.3
Banana bread (1 slice)	196	26	181	6.3
Cornbread (2-inch square)	180	24	333	7
Pancake (4-inch)	74	5	237	1
Pita, white (6-inch)	165	0	322	0.7
Corn tortilla (6-inch)	56	0	40	0.6
Flour tortilla (10-inch)	171	0	0	4.2
Waffle (7-inch)	218	52	383	10.6

WHAT'S THE BEST?

● Homemade. Storebought breakfast pastries and packaged baked goods such as muffins often contain dangerous trans fats. Make them at home with canola oil or another heart-friendly fat.

WHAT'S NOT SO GOOD?

● Exploding portions. A typical muffin tin or cupcake pan yields a 2-oz muffin—one that's about 2 3/4 inches in diameter and 2 inches high. Compare that to the gigantic muffins sold at bakeries.

● Refined flours. Choose whole-grain flours and meals for best nutrition; look for low-sugar baked goods, too.

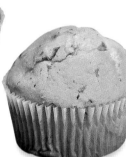

A muffin can be healthful enough if you make it yourself. But bought ready-made, it's likely to be laden with the danger fats— trans fats.

SATURATED FAT g	PROTEIN g	CARBOHYDRATE g	FIBER g	SUGARS g	GI
1.2	9	55	5.2	9.3	M
1.6	6	54	2.9	22.3	M
1.3	3	33	0.6	NA	H
1.3	4	25	2.3	NA	H
0.2	2	14	0.5	NA	NA
0.1	5	33	1.3	0.8	M
0.1	1	12	1.3	0.1	NA
0.9	4	30	1.7	0.9	NA
2.2	6	25	NA	NA	NA

PASTA

● ●

VERY LOW IN FAT
WHOLE WHEAT IS HIGH IN FIBER

Versatile and easy, pasta is a staple in most pantries.

WHAT'S IN IT?

Most pasta is made from enriched wheat flour, so it provides handsome amounts of folate, thiamin, riboflavin, niacin, iron, and selenium.

TIP

● Pasta often tastes better if it's cooked in salted water, though it will absorb some. One cup cooked in salted water supplies about 140mg of sodium, compared to 1.4mg cooked in unsalted water. Concerned about sodium? Add flavor with a squirt of lemon juice instead.

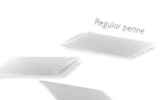

Regular penne

Spaghetti

STYLE 1 cup cooked	CALORIES	CHOLESTEROL mg	SODIUM mg	TOTAL FAT g
Regular (semolina)	197	0	1.4	0.9
Whole-wheat	174	0	4.2	0.8
Spinach or flavored	182	0	20	0.9
Homemade, w/egg (2 oz)	74	23	47	1
Fresh, storebought (2 oz)	75	19	3	0.6
Macaroni and cheese	390	10	730	17

*Pasta on its own in low in
fat and cholesterol, but adding
creamy sauces will pile on
the fat and calories.*

WHAT'S THE BEST?

● Whole-wheat pasta. One cup of cooked pasta supplies slightly over 2g fiber. The same amount of whole wheat has more than 6g.

● Vegetable or herb sauces. Opt for marinara, pesto, or a salsa cruda— chopped fresh tomatoes tossed with piping hot pasta—for best nutrition.

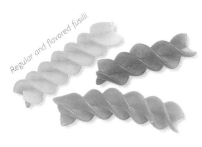

Regular and flavored fusilli

WHAT'S NOT SO GOOD?

● Boxed macaroni mixes and canned spaghetti marketed to children. These can contain 25 percent of the recommended daily limit of sodium for adults.

● Flavored pasta. They aren't bad for you, but don't think you're getting lots of extra vitamins if you choose spinach or tomato pasta—very little is actually added.

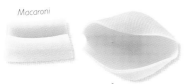

Macaroni

Pasta shell

SATURATED FAT g	PROTEIN g	CARBOHYDRATE g	FIBER g	SUGARS g	GI
0.1	7	40	2.4	2	L
0.1	7	37	6.3	1	L
0.1	6	37	NA	NA	NA
0.2	3	13	NA	NA	L
tr	3	14	NA	NA	NA
4	11	48	1	8	M

NOODLES

● ●

MOST ARE LOW IN FAT
SOME ARE GLUTEN-FREE

Pasta is usually made from hard wheat, but noodles can be made from the flour of a variety of grains and vegetables.

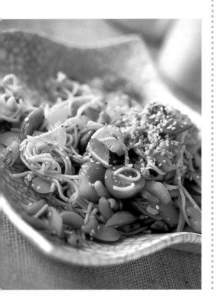

WHAT'S IN IT?

The nutrients vary depending on which grain or vegetable is used. As a general rule, however, most noodles are similar to pasta, rice, and other carbohydrate-dense foods.

TIP

● Be sure to read package directions—don't assume that Asian noodles should be cooked the same way that pasta is. Bean threads, for example, need to be soaked rather than boiled. (Soak them in very hot, not boiling, water; you may have to soak them a bit longer than directed.)

Noodles are often considered to be a healthy food, but beware—some can be high in sodium.

STYLE 1 cup cooked	CALORIES	CHOLESTEROL mg	SODIUM mg	TOTAL FAT g
Egg	213	53	11	2.4
Soba	113	0	68	0.1
Somen	231	0	283	0.3
Bean threads	190	0	0	0
Rice noodles	192	0	33	0.4
Chow mein	237	0	198	13.8

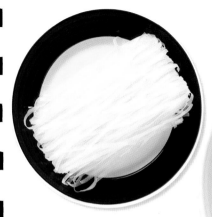

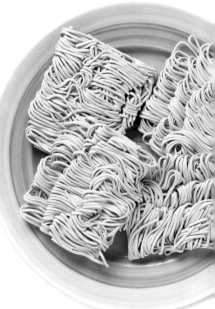

Look for rice noodles or egg noodles to use in recipes for Asian foods. Rice noodles are particularly healthful because they contain zero cholesterol and very little fat.

WHAT'S THE BEST?

● Cellophane noodles or bean threads (made with mung bean flour) and rice noodles are wheat-free and gluten-free. (Soba, made with buckwheat, often contain wheat.) If you're sensitive to wheat protein, look into these.

WHAT'S NOT SO GOOD?

● Ramen noodles. Whether they are sold in soup cups or in cellophane-wrapped blocks, these are best avoided. The noodles are "dried" by deep-frying and the seasoning packets contain very high amounts of sodium.

SATURATED FAT g	PROTEIN g	CARBOHYDRATE g	FIBER g	SUGARS g	GI
0.5	8	40	1.8	0.5	L
tr	6	24	NA	NA	NA
tr	7	49	NA	NA	NA
0	0	50	1	0	NA
tr	2	44	1.8	NA	NA
2	4	26	1.8	0.1	NA

RICE

● ●

LOW IN FAT AND CHOLESTEROL
GOOD SOURCE OF B VITAMINS

*R*ice is second only to wheat as the most cultivated grain in the world.

WHAT'S IN IT?

Rice provides thiamin, niacin, and vitamin B6, as well as magnesium, copper, and zinc. Choose brown rice and you'll get fiber, too.

TIP

● Wild rice is actually the seed of an aquatic grass. It has fewer calories and carbohydrate and more protein and fiber than white rice.

White long-grain rice

Wild rice

STYLE 1 cup cooked	CALORIES	CHOLESTEROL mg	SODIUM mg	TOTAL FAT g
Long-grain white	205	0	2	0.4
Glutinous or sticky	169	0	9	0.3
Long-grain brown	216	0	10	1.8
Wild	166	0	5	0.6
Packaged rice and pasta	246	2	1147	6
Instant white	162	0	5	0.3

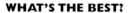

Cooked white rice

WHAT'S THE BEST?

● Brown rice. Higher in nutrients than white, brown rice has the bran intact. It can take up to 45 minutes to cook; look for quick and instant varieties to speed dinner preparations.

● Broth and juice. If plain rice tastes so bland that you reach for the butter dish or saltshaker to add flavor, try cooking rice in water mixed with broth or vegetable juice.

Rich in vitamins and minerals, and low in sodium and fat, white rice is usually quick to cook, too.

WHAT'S NOT SO GOOD?

● Packaged flavored rice, or rice-and-pasta mixes. One cup can contain nearly 1,200mg of sodium—about half of the recommended daily allowance.

● Rinsing rice. Most is enriched, and the added nutrients sit on the surface. When you rinse the rice, the nutrients go down the drain. (Some imported rices should be rinsed, though; check package labels.)

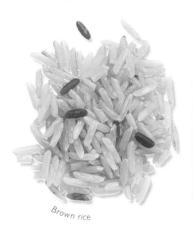

Brown rice

SATURATED FAT g	PROTEIN g	CARBOHYDRATE g	FIBER g	SUGARS g	GI
0.1	4	45	0.6	0.3	M
tr	4	37	1.7	0.1	H
0.4	5	45	3.5	0.5	L
0.4	7	35	3	1.1	L
1	5	43	2	6	H
tr	3	35	0.9	2	H

CEREALS AND GRAINS

● ● ●

HIGH IN FIBER, VITAMINS, AND MINERALS

If you're stuck in a rice or pasta rut, break out of it! You'll find a variety of grains in supermarkets and natural foods stores.

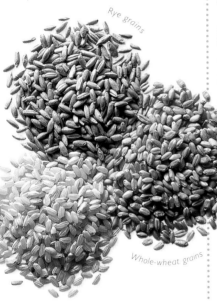

Rye grains

Whole-wheat grains

WHAT'S IN IT?

Some grains supply high-quality vegetable protein as well as fiber and complex carbohydrates. They also provide B vitamins and trace minerals.

TIP

● For best quality, buy small amounts; stores with high turnover will have fresher grains. In addition to the varieties below, you may see teff and sorghum, which are types of millet, and spelt or kamut, which are related to wheat. Rye and triticale, a hybrid of wheat and rye, are rarely available in any form but flour.

STYLE 1 cup cooked	CALORIES	CHOLESTEROL mg	SODIUM mg	TOTAL FAT g
Cornmeal (polenta)	110	0	11	1.1
Grits, quick cooking	145	0	0	0.5
Millet	207	0	3	1.7
Quinoa	159	0	9	2.5
Buckwheat groats	155	0	7	1

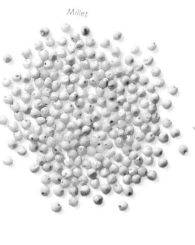

Millet

WHAT'S THE BEST?

● Whole grains are digested slowly and have less of an effect on blood sugar levels than processed and refined grains.

WHAT'S NOT SO GOOD?

● Be wary of buying grains sold in clear containers. Exposure to heat or sunlight can cause nutrient loss.

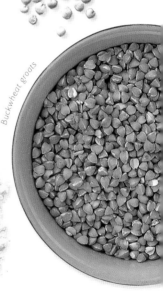

Buckwheat groats

Cornmeal

SATURATED FAT g	PROTEIN g	CARBOHYDRATE g	FIBER g	SUGARS g	GI
0.2	1	23	2.2	0	NA
tr	3	31	0.5	0.2	NA
0.3	6	41	2.2	0.7	NA
0.3	6	29	2.5	NA	NA
tr	6	33	4.5	2.2	L

BREAKFAST CEREALS AND CEREAL BARS

● ●

CAN BE HIGH IN SUGARS
AND TRANS FATS

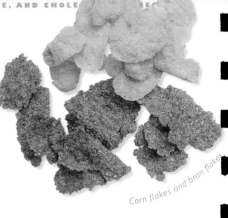

Corn flakes and bran flakes

They look so nutritious, with their photographs of wheat or corn and fresh fruit, and banners proclaiming "cholesterol-free!" But what's inside those boxes of cereal?

WHAT'S IN IT?

Most cereals are fortified with a host of vitamins and minerals, as a quick scan of the Nutrition Facts label shows. Few are high in fiber, most are high in added sugar, and some are high in trans fats.

TIPS

● Cereal with added fruit is rarely a nutritional bargain—it's a small amount of fruit, and it usually comes with a hefty amount of added sugars. Buy plain cereals and add your own fruit.

● The vitamins in fortified cereal often leach into the milk, so it's important to drink all of the milk for full nutritional benefits.

STYLE 1 cup, without milk	CALORIES	CHOLESTEROL mg	SODIUM mg	TOTAL FAT g
Corn flakes	101	0	203	0.2
Oat circles	111	0	273	1.8
Wheat flakes	107	0	218	1
Crispy rice	111	0	206	0.1
Chocolate-flavored corn puffs	117	0	171	1
Wheat flakes with raisins	188	0	350	1.5
Bran cereal (½ cup)	81	0	80	1
Puffed wheat	44	0	1	0.1
Raisin granola bar (1½ oz)	193	1	121	7.7

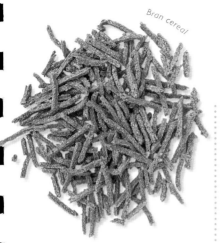

Bran cereal

WHAT'S NOT SO GOOD?

● Refined flours. Scan cereal box labels as you would bread labels and opt for those with "100% whole" grains. Yes, cereals made with refined flours often feature added vitamins and minerals, but they're not fortified with fiber.

● Crunch. Often cereals with "crunchy nuggets" or crispy textures are made with trans fats.

WHAT'S THE BEST?

● Simplicity. When it comes to cereal, the simpler the better. Brief ingredients lists mean fewer sweeteners, fewer trans fats, and fewer artificial colors.

● High fiber. Although some bran cereals supply as many as 10g of fiber per 1/2 cup, 3g is an acceptable lower limit.

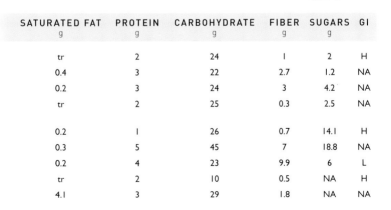

Cereal bar

SATURATED FAT g	PROTEIN g	CARBOHYDRATE g	FIBER g	SUGARS g	GI
tr	2	24	1	2	H
0.4	3	22	2.7	1.2	NA
0.2	3	24	3	4.2	NA
tr	2	25	0.3	2.5	NA
0.2	1	26	0.7	14.1	H
0.3	5	45	7	18.8	NA
0.2	4	23	9.9	6	L
tr	2	10	0.5	NA	H
4.1	3	29	1.8	NA	NA

WHEAT AND ITS PRODUCTS

● ● ●

EXCELLENT SOURCE OF FIBER, VITAMINS, AND MINERALS

*M*ost wheat is ground down to make flour, but some is left whole and can be served either as a breakfast cereal or as a side dish.

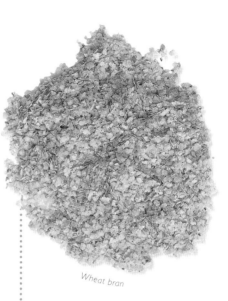

Wheat bran

TIP

● Wheat berries have an appealing texture and wonderfully nutty flavor, but they require lengthy cooking— at least 1 hour—or presoaking to become edible. Bulgur and cracked wheat have the same flavor and similar texture and cook in less time.

WHAT'S IN IT?

Wheat contains ample amounts of soluble and insoluble fiber, iron, and protein. Its bran and germ contain phytochemicals such as lignans, plant compounds that may reduce the risk for some cancers and for heart disease. Different wheat products contain different nutrients, but hard wheat supplies niacin, magnesium, thiamin, vitamin B6, folate, riboflavin, phosphorus, and zinc.

STYLE 1 cup cooked	CALORIES	CHOLESTEROL mg	SODIUM mg	TOTAL FAT g
Wheat berries	84	0	1	0.4
Bulgur	151	0	9	0.4
Couscous	176	0	8	0.3
Farina	117	0	0	0.2
Wheat germ (2 tbsp)	52	0	2	1.4
Wheat bran (2 tbsp)	16	0	0	0.3

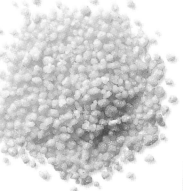

Couscous

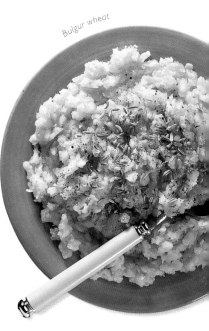

Bulgur wheat

Made from wheat kernels, Bulgur wheat is a good source of bran and germ.

WHAT'S THE BEST?

● Wheat germ and wheat bran. These are different—the germ, or embryo, contains generous amounts of folate, vitamin E, B vitamins, and fiber; the bran, or outer covering of the grain, contains even more fiber. Sprinkle over cereal or yogurt, or use in lieu of breadcrumbs in meatloaf or as a coating for foods to be sautéed (watch the heat, though, as these may burn more easily). Or use in baked goods—for each cup of white flour, replace up to ¼ cup of the flour with wheat germ.

WHAT'S NOT SO GOOD?

● Poor storage. It doesn't contain much fat, but whole wheat (particularly the germ) does contain some and can become rancid. Refrigerate or freeze whole-grain products to maintain their freshness; bring them to room temperature before using.

SATURATED FAT g	PROTEIN g	CARBOHYDRATE g	FIBER g	SUGARS g	GI
tr	4	20	3	NA	NA
tr	6	34	8.2	0.2	L
tr	6	36	2.2	0.2	M
tr	3	25	3.3	3	NA
0.2	3	7	1.8	1.2	M
0.1	1	5	3.2	0.2	M

BARLEY AND ITS PRODUCTS

● ● ●

HIGH IN SOLUBLE FIBER

*M*ost of the barley grown today goes to breweries and distilleries, but not all. Serve it as a side dish or add it to soups.

Rich in minerals, pearled barley has a chewy texture that makes it a good addition to hearty soups.

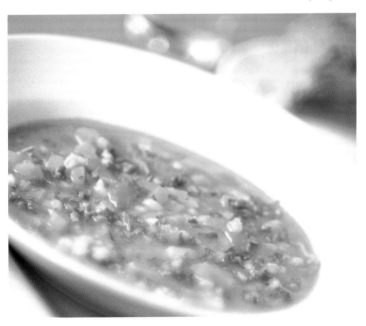

STYLE 1 cup cooked	CALORIES	CHOLESTEROL mg	SODIUM mg	TOTAL FAT g
Pearled	193	0	5	0.7
Hulled	270	0	1	2

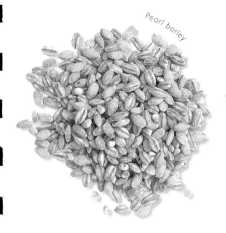

Pearl barley

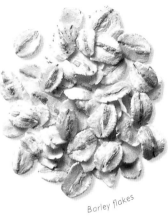

Barley flakes

WHAT'S IN IT?

Barley is an excellent source of niacin, iron, and selenium, as well as fiber. It provides some thiamin and vitamin B6.

WHAT'S THE BEST?

⬤ Unless you shop at a natural foods store, you might have trouble finding any form of barley other than pearled. It's also available in flakes (they have a texture similar to rolled oats), barley grits, or quick-cooking.

⬤ Hulled barley still has the germ and most of the bran, so it's the most nutrient-rich form of barley. However, it needs to be soaked for several hours before cooking, and it can take an hour or so to cook.

WHAT'S NOT SO GOOD?

⬤ If it's barley's pleasantly chewy texture you love, take the 45 minutes or so to make pearled barley. Quick-cooking barley can be on the table in much less time, but it lacks the hearty texture.

TIP

⬤ Pearled barley, sometimes just called pearl barley, is not a whole grain; its bran has been removed. Hulled barley does contain the bran. Still, 1 cup of cooked pearled barley supplies a generous 6g fiber.

SATURATED FAT g	PROTEIN g	CARBOHYDRATE g	FIBER g	SUGARS g	GI
0.1	4	44	6	0.4	L
tr	7	59	14	NA	L

OATS AND ITS PRODUCTS

● ● ●

EXCELLENT SOURCE OF FIBER

Of all the cereal grains and grasses, oats are the most nutritious. They retain most of their nutrients after hulling (a process that removes a grain's outer, inedible coating) because the bran and germ are not removed. Only further refining removes the bran and germ.

TIP

● Rolled oats and quick oats are interchangeable in recipes, though you'll taste a difference in texture if you eat them as cereal. Rolled oats take slightly longer to cook, but many think they are worth the few extra minutes.

WHAT'S IN IT?

Oats provide more protein than bulgur and brown rice, as well as thiamin, iron, selenium, and fiber, half of which is cholesterol-lowering soluble fiber.

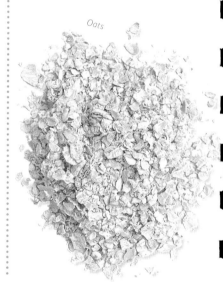

Oats

STYLE 3-oz	CALORIES	CHOLESTEROL mg	SODIUM mg	TOTAL FAT g
Oats (regular, quick, or instant)	109	0	2	1.8
Oat bran (1 cup)	88	0	2	1.9
Instant, plain (1 packet)	97	0	80	1.7
Instant, cinnamon & spice	177	0	280	1.9

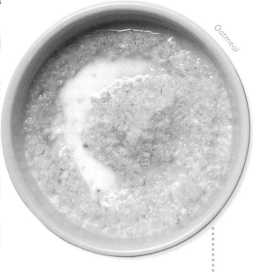

Oatmeal

For a breakfast that packs a nutritional punch (protein, minerals, and fiber), make your own oatmeal.

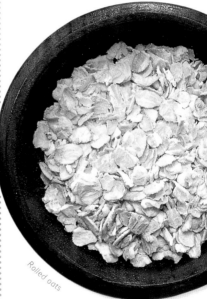

Rolled oats

WHAT'S THE BEST?

❋ Oats also contain saponins, a group of phytochemicals that appear to regulate blood flow.

WHAT'S NOT SO GOOD?

❋ Instant oatmeal packets. High in sugar and sodium, these are best left on the supermarket shelf. Make a bowl of rolled oats—use milk for a boost of flavor and calcium—and stir in cinnamon or cut-up fruit.

❋ Long cooking times. If your mornings are hectic, make oatmeal overnight in a slow cooker.

SATURATED FAT g	PROTEIN g	CARBOHYDRATE g	FIBER g	SUGARS g	GI
0.3	5	19	3	0.9	M
0.4	7	25	5.7	NA	M
0.3	4	17	3	0	M
0.4	5	35	2.6	15.5	NA

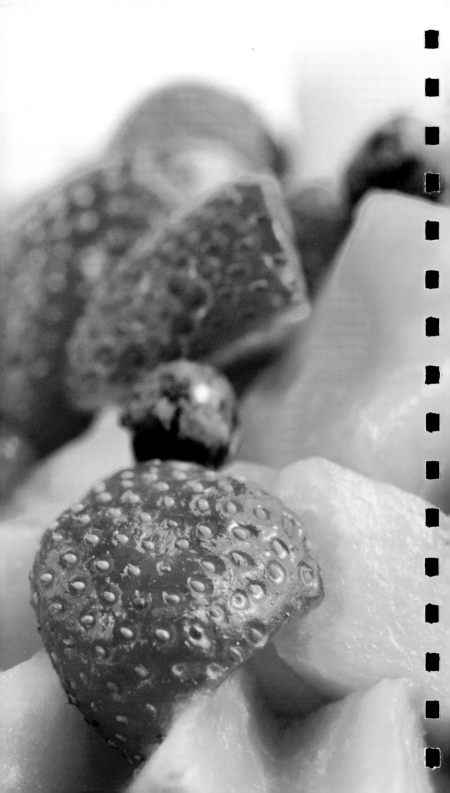

FRUIT AND VEGETABLES

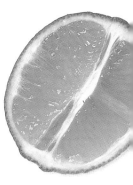

You'll be hard pressed to find anyone who can fault fruits and vegetables. Not only do these foods provide an array of vitamins, quite a few minerals, and fiber, but they also contain phytochemicals, compounds, and pigments that can promote health in dramatic ways. Research indicates that these compounds have antioxidant properties that can keep cells healthy, reduce levels of LDL *("bad") cholesterol and boost levels of* HDL *("good") cholesterol, and protect against different cancers and heart disease. Some researchers, in fact, wonder if these can actually reverse the effects of aging.*

As a general rule, deeply colored fruits and vegetables contain higher levels of the beneficial pigments, but paler foods often contain different compounds (some antioxidants and phytochemicals are colorless). Eat a variety of produce in a rainbow of colors for best nutrition.

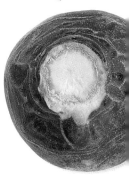

POPULAR FRUITS

● ● ●

FULL OF FIBER. SOME ARE HIGHER
IN NUTRIENTS THAN OTHERS

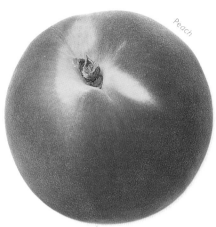

Peach

Whether you slice a peach over your cereal for breakfast, grab an apple for a snack, or have stewed pears for dessert, fruits are easy to incorporate into eating plans.

Grapes

Plums

WHAT'S IN IT?

In general, fruits contain varying amounts of vitamins, especially C and A. Most fruits are high in fiber, most of which is soluble—the type that helps to reduce blood cholesterol levels. Fruits also contain phytochemicals, plant compounds and pigments that contain antioxidants and can protect from a variety of diseases.

STYLE 1 medium, raw, w/skin	CALORIES	CHOLESTEROL mg	SODIUM mg	TOTAL FAT g
Apple	81	0	0	0.5
Pear	98	0	0	0.7
Peach	42	0	0	tr
Nectarine	67	0	0	0.6
Apricot	17	0	tr	0.1
Plum	36	0	0	0.4
Cherries (10)	43	0	0	0.1
Grapes, green or red (10)	36	0	1	0.3

Ripen fruits at room temperature, but then store them in the refrigerator to maintain flavor and freshness.

WHAT'S THE BEST?

Dark or deep colors. Red or black grapes are higher in nutrients than green grapes, and cherries and plums tend to have higher concentrations of beneficial compounds than do pears and apples.

Variety. Just because green grapes, pears, and apples aren't as high in vitamins as some other fruits doesn't mean they're nutritionally bankrupt. One apple provides almost 4g fiber as well as flavonoids. Green grapes provide different benefits than do red ones.

WHAT'S NOT SO GOOD?

Juice. High in sugars and very low in fiber, juice and cider come up short compared to the fruit.

Peeled fruit, particularly apples. Pigments are concentrated in the skin. Discard the peel and you discard the antioxidants. Peels also provide fiber, vitamins, and minerals.

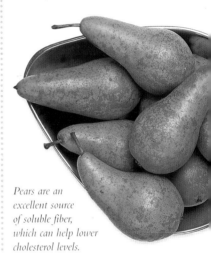

Pears are an excellent source of soluble fiber, which can help lower cholesterol levels.

SATURATED FAT g	PROTEIN g	CARBOHYDRATE g	FIBER g	SUGARS g	GI
tr	0.3	21	3.7	18	L
tr	0.6	25	4	17	L
tr	0.7	11	2	8	L
tr	1.3	16	2.2	12	L
tr	0.5	4	0.8	3	M
tr	0.5	9	1	5	L
tr	0.7	11	1.4	8.7	L
tr	0.3	9	0.5	7	L

CITRUS FRUITS

● ● ●

HIGH IN VITAMIN C AND FIBER

In addition to the common citrus fruits, you may find blood oranges, kumquats, and hybrids like pummelos, tangelos, and even ugli fruit in your market.

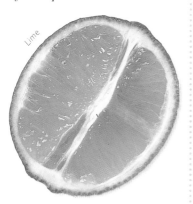

Lime

WHAT'S IN IT?

Best known for their high vitamin C content, citrus fruits also supply generous amounts of folate, fiber, and some carotenoids, or plant pigments.

TIP

● Unlike other citrus fruits where the pulp is eaten, lemon and lime are mostly consumed as juice (though sometimes a slice or wedge gets eaten), which is why only juice for these fruits is included below. Don't forget the zest, or colored outer part of the peel, which is high in carotenoids and other compounds.

STYLE 1 medium, unless noted	CALORIES	CHOLESTEROL mg	SODIUM mg	TOTAL FAT g
Orange	62	0	0	0.2
Tangerine	37	0	1	0.2
Mandarin, canned (1 cup)	154	0	15	0.3
Grapefruit, pink or red (½ med)	52	0	0	0.2
Grapefruit, white (½ med)	39	0	0	0.1
Lemon (1, juice only)	12	0	1	0
Lime (1, juice only)	10	0	tr	tr
Orange juice (1 cup)	112	0	2	0.5

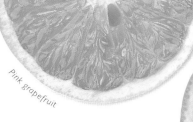

Pink grapefruit

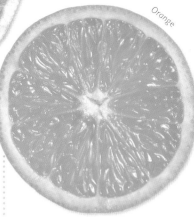

Orange

WHAT'S THE BEST?

● Different citrus fruits provide different nutritional benefits. Oranges and tangerines are high in beta cryptoxanthin, a pigment in the carotenoid family that can inhibit the growth of some tumors; pink and red grapefruit supply lycopene, another carotenoid pigment that can protect against prostate and other cancers; and all citrus fruits contain limonene compounds, which are thought to neutralize some cancer-causing chemicals.

Rich in vitamin C they may be, but citrus fruits are also packed with cancer-fighting compounds.

WHAT'S NOT SO GOOD?

● Processed fruit. Juice lacks fiber, and if you've been tempted to buy jars of peeled orange or grapefruit sections with the membranes cut away, think twice. Many of the beneficial compounds are found in the pith, the white part of the peel.

● Lightweight fruit. Citrus fruit that feels heavy for its size will be juicier than those that feel lighter.

SATURATED FAT g	PROTEIN g	CARBOHYDRATE g	FIBER g	SUGARS g	GI
tr	1	15	3.1	12.2	L
tr	1	9	1.9	7.5	NA
tr	1	41	1.8	39	M
tr	1	13	1.9	8.5	L
tr	1	10	1.3	8.6	L
0	tr	4	0.2	1.1	NA
tr	tr	3	0.2	0.6	NA
tr	2	26	0.5	20.8	M

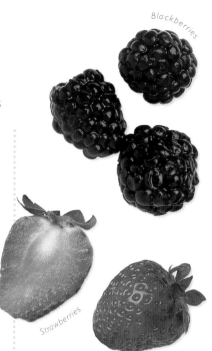

Blackberries

BERRIES

● ● ●

HIGH IN VITAMINS AND ANTIOXIDANTS

When researchers made a list of the most healthful fresh fruits and vegetables, high-in-antioxidant blueberries and blackberries held the top two positions; strawberries came in at number four.

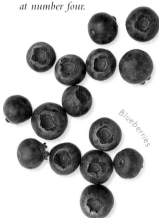

Strawberries

Blueberries

WHAT'S IN IT?

Just about all berries are low in calories yet high in fiber, and nearly all are sky-high in antioxidant phytochemicals and vitamins. Most are potent sources of vitamin C. Ounce for ounce, strawberries are higher in vitamin C than oranges.

STYLE 1 cup	CALORIES	CHOLESTEROL mg	SODIUM mg	TOTAL FAT g
Blueberries	83	0	1	0.5
Blackberries	62	0	1	0.7
Raspberries	64	0	1	0.8
Cranberries	44	0	2	0.1
Strawberries	43	0	1	0.5
Gooseberries	66	0	2	0.9
Red currants	63	0	1	0.2

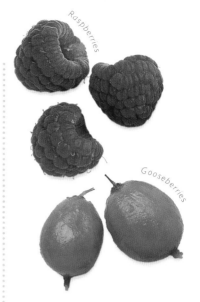

Raspberries

Gooseberries

WHAT'S THE BEST?

All blue, red, and deep purplish berries are high in anthocyanins, plant pigments that can protect against some cancers, preserve eyesight, and prevent heart disease.

Silvery blueberries. Don't shun berries with a whitish coating. It's called bloom, and it actually protects them. (Grapes and plums can have bloom, too.)

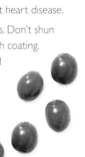

Cranberries

WHAT'S NOT SO GOOD?

Short seasons. Fresh, locally grown berries are available just briefly, and cranberries in particular can be hard to find from January through September. Fortunately, cranberries freeze well, so buy a few extra bags to stick in the freezer.

Cooked berries. Vitamin C breaks down when exposed to heat, so for best nutrition, eat berries raw or sprinkled on cereal or yogurt, rather than baked into pies or muffins.

SATURATED FAT g	PROTEIN g	CARBOHYDRATE g	FIBER g	SUGARS g	GI
tr	1	21	3.5	14.4	NA
tr	2	14	7.6	7	NA
tr	1	15	8.0	5.4	NA
tr	tr	12	4.3	3.8	NA
tr	1	10	3.3	9	L
tr	1	15	6.5	NA	NA
tr	2	15	4.8	8.3	NA

TROPICAL AND EXOTIC FRUITS

● ● ●

ALMOST ALL ARE RICH IN
VITAMIN C AND FIBER

If pineapple and melon are the extent of your tropical fruit forays, expand your horizons. Most supermarkets sell a wide assortment.

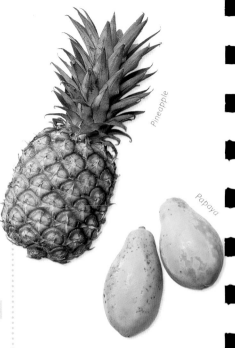

Pineapple

Papaya

TIP

● Make it your goal to buy one unusual fruit every week. If you've no idea whether the peel or seeds are edible or even how to peel and seed it, consult a general cookbook or check the Internet.

WHAT'S IN IT?

Guavas, kiwifruit, mango, and papaya are high in vitamin C and fiber; watermelon provides 40 percent more lycopene per ounce than raw tomatoes.

STYLE 1 medium, unless noted	CALORIES	CHOLESTEROL mg	SODIUM mg	TOTAL FAT g
Banana	109	0	1	0.6
Honeydew (⅛ med)	56	0	16	0.2
Cantaloupe (⅛ med)	24	0	6	0.2
Watermelon (1/16 med)	92	0	6	1
Pineapple (1 cup, diced)	76	0	2	0.7
Guava	46	0	3	0.5
Papaya	119	0	9	0.4
Mango	135	0	4	0.6
Kiwifruit	46	0	4	0.3
Carambola (star fruit)	30	0	2	0.3
Pomegranate	105	0	6	0.5

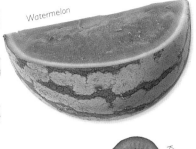

Watermelon

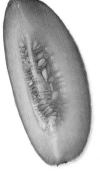

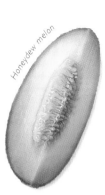

Honeydew melon

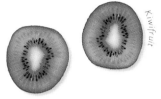

Kiwifruit

WHAT'S THE BEST?

● Variety and color. Honeydew, for example, doesn't contain lycopene like watermelon or beta carotene like cantaloupe, but it is a good source of two carotenoids called lutein and zeaxanthin, which can protect against age-related eye disorders. Kiwi also contains these compounds.

WHAT'S NOT SO GOOD?

● Skip the precut melon at the supermarket. Vitamin C breaks down rapidly when exposed to oxygen, but the rind protects this vitamin—and maintains freshness and flavor.

● Unwashed fruit. Even though you don't eat melon rind, bacteria on it can be transferred to the melon's flesh when you cut the fruit.

SATURATED FAT g	PROTEIN g	CARBOHYDRATE g	FIBER g	SUGARS g	GI
0.2	1	28	2.8	18	L
tr	1	15	1	13	NA
tr	1	6	0.6	7	NA
0.1	2	21	1.4	19	H
tr	1	19	1.9	18	M
0.2	1	11	4.9	6	NA
0.1	2	30	5.5	18	M
0.1	1	35	3.8	31	M
tr	1	12	2.6	8	M
tr	1	7	1.5	4.7	NA
tr	1	26	0.9	25.5	NA

DRIED FRUITS

● ●

CONCENTRATED SOURCE
OF NUTRIENTS

*H*igh in fiber and many minerals but also high in sugars and calories, dried fruit is best eaten in small amounts.

TIP

● Sulfur dioxide is often added to golden raisins and light-colored dried fruit to maintain the pale colors. If you are sensitive to sulfites, read labels carefully. Natural foods stores are more likely to carry unsulfured dried fruit.

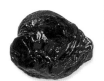

WHAT'S IN IT?

Raisins and dried plums are high in fiber, iron, and potassium. Figs provide some vitamin E and B6.

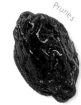

Prunes

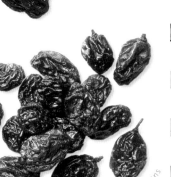

Raisins

STYLE ¼ cup	CALORIES	CHOLESTEROL mg	SODIUM mg	TOTAL FAT g
Dates	122	0	1	0.2
Dried plums (prunes)	102	0	2	0.2
Raisins	109	0	4	0.2
Golden raisins	109	0	4	0.2
Zante currants	102	0	3	0.1
Figs	127	0	5	0.6
Apricot halves	78	0	3	0.2

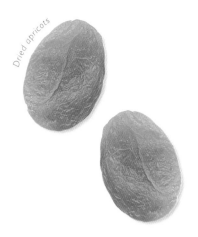

Dried apricots

WHAT'S NOT SO GOOD?

● Tooth decay. Because they are so sticky, dried fruits can remain on and around teeth long after eating, increasing the risk for cavities.

WHAT'S THE BEST?

● Small portions. Because dried fruits are high in sugars, they're best consumed in very limited amounts amounts. Rather than snacking on handful after handful, toss a tablespoon or two into a salad, or add to sautéed greens.

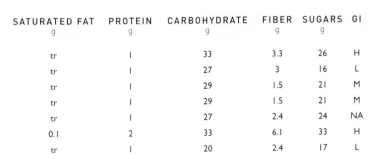

Dates

Dates are very high in sugars, so don't make the mistake of assuming they make a good alternative to candy.

SATURATED FAT g	PROTEIN g	CARBOHYDRATE g	FIBER g	SUGARS g	GI
tr	1	33	3.3	26	H
tr	1	27	3	16	L
tr	1	29	1.5	21	M
tr	1	29	1.5	21	M
tr	1	27	2.4	24	NA
0.1	2	33	6.1	33	H
tr	1	20	2.4	17	L

SHOOTS, STALKS, AND LEAVES

● ● ●

INCREDIBLY HIGH IN A
VARIETY OF NUTRIENTS

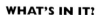

Red cabbage

With a minimum number of calories and a maximum amount of vitamins, minerals, and disease-fighting chemicals, these vegetables are nutritional superstars.

WHAT'S IN IT?

Calcium (266mg in a cup of collards), iron (2mg in chard), vitamin C (101mg in broccoli), vitamin A (17,707 IU in kale), and folate (268mcg in asparagus).

TIP

● Some of these vegetables—cabbage, kale, and Brussels sprouts in particular—are at their best in winter, long after most vegetables have peaked.

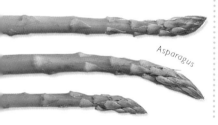

Asparagus

STYLE 1/2 cup cooked, unless noted	CALORIES	CHOLESTEROL mg	SODIUM mg	TOTAL FAT g
Asparagus (or 6 spears)	22	0	10	0.3
Broccoli, chopped	28	0	32	0.3
Celery (1 med stalk, raw)	6	0	35	tr
Collards (1 cup)	49	0	30	0.7
Chard (1 cup)	35	0	313	0.1
Kale (1 cup)	36	0	30	0.5
Cauliflower, chopped	14	0	9	0.3
Red cabbage	16	0	6	0.2
Brussels sprouts	28	0	16	0.4
Bok choy (1 cup)	20	0	58	0.3
Artichoke (1 med.)	60	0	114	0.2
Green beans	22	0	2	0.2

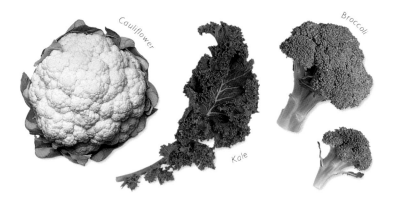

Cauliflower

Kale

Broccoli

WHAT'S THE BEST?

● Crucifers. Members of the cabbage family—broccoli, collards, kale, cauliflower, Brussels sprouts, and bok choy—contain antioxidant vitamins, minerals, and potent phytochemicals.

● Asparagus is a distant relative of the onion family and contains smaller amounts of their powerful sulfur compounds.

WHAT'S NOT SO GOOD?

● Overcooking. Sulfur compounds in many of these vegetables are what make them so healthful, and what gives them their unpleasant aromas. Cook them briefly to lessen the smell.

● Boiling. Nutrients leach into the water and unless you reuse the cooking liquid in soups, they're dumped down the drain. Keep vitamins in the food by roasting or sautéing.

SATURATED FAT g	PROTEIN g	CARBOHYDRATE g	FIBER g	SUGARS g	GI
tr	2	4	1.4	1.4	L
tr	2	6	2.6	1	L
tr	0.3	1.5	0.7	0.4	L
tr	4	9	5.3	0.8	L
tr	3	7	3.7	1.9	L
tr	2	7	2.6	1.6	L
tr	1	3	1.7	0.9	L
tr	1	3	1.5	2.1	L
tr	2	6	2	1.4	L
tr	3	3	1.7	1.4	L
tr	4	13	6.6	3.3	L
0	1	5	2	1.4	L

ROOTS, BULBS, AND STARCHY VEGETABLES

● ● ●

CONCENTRATED SOURCE
OF NUTRIENTS

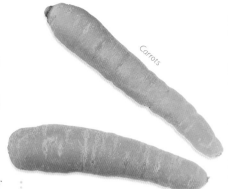

Carrots

These come from a variety of botanical families: carrots and parsnips are related to parsley; sweet potatoes to morning glories; and rutabaga, radishes, kohlrabi, and turnips are cruciferous vegetables, the same family that gives cabbage, broccoli, kale, and collards their nutritional benefits. Potatoes are a member of the nightshade family.

WHAT'S IN IT?

Roots and tubers are high in carbohydrates, which provide energy and nutrients for growing plants.

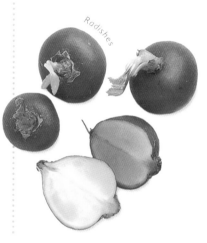

Radishes

STYLE 1 cup cooked, unless noted	CALORIES	CHOLESTEROL mg	SODIUM mg	TOTAL FAT g
Carrots	55	0	90	0.2
Carrot (1 large, raw)	30	0	50	0.1
Fennel (raw)	27	0	45	0.2
Radishes, sliced (½ cup, raw)	9	0	23	tr
Turnips, cubed	34	0	30	0.1
Jicama, sliced (raw)	46	0	5	0.1

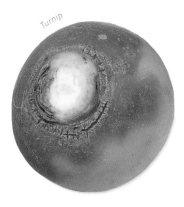

Turnip

WHAT'S THE BEST?

● Cooked vegetables. Many of these vegetables have tough cell walls. Cooking breaks them down and increases the availability of the nutrients within.

TIP

● As with other fruits and vegetables, roots and tubers with deeper colors tend to be higher in nutrients. Carrots and sweet potatoes are high in carotenoids and beets in anthocyanins, the same beneficial pigments that make blueberries so healthy.

WHAT'S NOT SO GOOD?

● Large vegetables. Roots and tubers tend to be tougher and more fibrous than other vegetables, and larger ones tend to be tougher than smaller ones.

● Rich toppings. These vegetables are high in a variety of nutrients and can be surprisingly low in calories. Keep the cream sauces off the corn and the butter sauce off the carrots—and both out of the mashed potatoes —except for occasional meals.

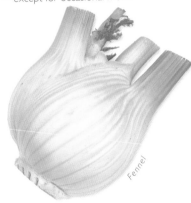

Fennel

SATURATED FAT g	PROTEIN g	CARBOHYDRATE g	FIBER g	SUGARS g	GI
tr	2	13	4.7	5.4	H
tr	1	7	2.2	3.3	H
NA	1	6	2.7	NA	NA
tr	0.4	2	0.9	1.2	L
tr	1	8	3.1	4.7	NA
tr	1	11	5.9	2.2	NA

ROOTS, BULBS, AND STARCHY VEGETABLES

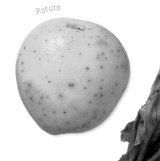

Potato

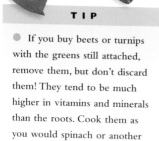

Sweet potato

Beets

TIP

● If you buy beets or turnips with the greens still attached, remove them, but don't discard them! They tend to be much higher in vitamins and minerals than the roots. Cook them as you would spinach or another cooking green.

WHAT'S IN IT?

● Potatoes are fairly high in vitamin C, but this nutrient breaks down when it is exposed to heat. You're better off planning to get your C from other foods.

STYLE 1 cup cooked, unless noted	CALORIES	CHOLESTEROL mg	SODIUM mg	TOTAL FAT g
Potato, baked, w/skin (1 med)	163	0	12	0.3
Potato, mashed, w/milk	174	4	63	1.2
Sweet potato, baked (1 med)	103	0	41	0.2
Beets, sliced (½ cup)	37	0	65	0.2
Parsnips, sliced (½ cup)	55	0	8	0.2
Corn (½ cup)	89	0	14	1
Rutabaga, cubed	66	0	34	0.4
Kohlrabi	48	0	35	0.2

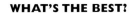

Parsnips

WHAT'S THE BEST?

● Roasting. These vegetables
are comparatively high in
sugars, which caramelize at
high temperatures. Make the
most of their natural sweetness by
scrubbing, cutting into 1-inch chunks,
arranging on a baking sheet in a single
layer (drizzle with olive oil and sprinkle
with salt), and then roasting in a 400°F
oven until browned and tender.

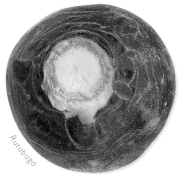

Rutabaga

WHAT'S NOT SO GOOD?

● French fries. Potatoes are the
most-consumed vegetable in the
United States, and the vast majority
of those are deep-fried. Instead of
French fries, choose baked, roasted,
or mashed potatoes (reserve some
of the water they were cooked in and
use it instead of some of the cream
or milk when mashing).

SATURATED FAT g	PROTEIN g	CARBOHYDRATE g	FIBER g	SUGARS g	GI
tr	4	35	3.6	3	H
0.7	4	37	3.2	3.2	H
tr	2	24	3.8	9.6	L
tr	1	8	1.7	6.8	NA
tr	1	13	2.8	3.7	NA
0.2	3	21	2.3	2.1	NA
tr	2	15	3	10.2	NA
tr	3	11	1.8	4.6	NA

VEGETABLE FRUITS

NUTRIENT-RICH

*A*ll *but one of the foods in this section are botanically fruits but are cooked as vegetables. Rhubarb is actually a vegetable.*

TIP

● Avocado connoisseurs prefer Hass, the smaller of the two common commercial varieties. Hass avocados have dark green, almost black, pebbly skin and a rich, succulent texture. They are higher in folate, iron, and vitamin E than Fuerte avocados, the larger, bright green ones.

WHAT'S IN IT?

Red and yellow bell peppers contain about twice as much vitamin C as green bell peppers; red ones are also high in carotenoids.

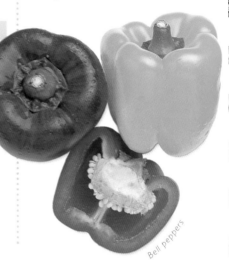

Bell peppers

STYLE 1 cup cooked, unless noted	CALORIES	CHOLESTEROL mg	SODIUM mg	TOTAL FAT g
Hass avocado (½ med, raw)	153	0	10	15
Pumpkin	49	0	2	0.2
Cucumber, sliced (raw)	14	0	2	0.1
Dill pickle (1 med)	12	0	833	0.1
Zucchini, sliced	29	0	5	0.1
Acorn squash, cubed	115	0	8	0.3
Bell pepper, red or green (1 med)	32	0	2	0.2
Jalapeño pepper (1 raw)	4	0	0.1	tr

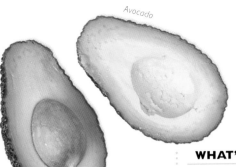

Avocado

WHAT'S THE BEST?

● Variety. Olives and avocados supply heart-healthy fats; tomatoes, zucchini, cucumbers, pumpkin, and squash contain a variety of carotenoids; bell peppers have vitamin C and hotter peppers capsaicin, an antioxidant that may protect against cancers and help prevent blood clots.

● Skin. Some foods—cucumbers, eggplant, and zucchini among them— have pale flesh but deeply colored peels. Be sure to eat the skins of these foods, since that is where the beneficial plant pigments are found.

WHAT'S NOT SO GOOD?

● Burns. Jalapeños and other hot peppers get their heat from capsaicin, a substance that can actually cause blisters. Protect yourself by wearing gloves when chopping, and by serving very spicy foods with dairy (milk contains a protein that neutralizes capsaicin). Most of a pepper's capsaicin is in the white ribs and seeds. Removing them can reduce the heat by as much as 90 percent.

Zucchini

SATURATED FAT g	PROTEIN g	CARBOHYDRATE g	FIBER g	SUGARS g	GI
2.2	2	6	4.2	0.3	NA
tr	2	12	2.7	2.5	NA
tr	1	2	0.8	2.4	NA
tr	0.4	3	0.8	2.3	NA
tr	1	7	2.5	3	NA
tr	2	30	9	NA	NA
tr	1	8	2.1	3	L
tr	0.2	0.8	0.4	0.5	NA

VEGETABLE FRUITS

Olives

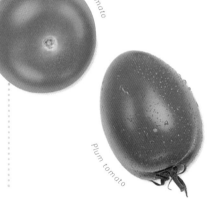

Tomato

Plum tomato

WHAT'S IN IT?

Olives are high in monounsaturated fats and vitamin E, but did you know that they are high in iron, too? Six super-colossal black olives supply almost 40 percent of the daily value for this mineral. (They also contain about one third of the recommended limit of sodium.)

TIP

● Most fruits should be ripened at room temperature and then refrigerated, but not tomatoes. Exposure to temperatures below 55°F prevents their flavor from developing and can give them a mealy texture.

STYLE 1 cup cooked, unless noted	CALORIES	CHOLESTEROL mg	SODIUM mg	TOTAL FAT g
Rhubarb (cooked w/sugar)	278	0	2	0.1
Rhubarb (raw)	26	0	5	0.2
Olives, Spanish w/ pimento (5)	30	0	190	2.5
Okra (½ cup)	26	0	4	0.1
Eggplant, cubed	28	0	3	0.2
Tomato (1 med, raw)	26	0	11	0.4
Tomatoes, stewed	80	0	460	2.7

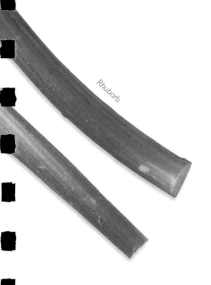

Rhubarb

WHAT'S NOT SO GOOD?

● Rhubarb. A good source of vitamin C on its own, this is invariably cooked with large amounts of sugar. Some chutney or relish recipes tame its astringency with a minimum of sugar and are worth seeking out.

WHAT'S THE BEST?

● Cooked tomatoes. Tomatoes are high in lycopene, a carotenoid that can reduce the risk of heart attacks and of cancers of the digestive tract. Cooking and canning concentrates the lycopene in tomatoes.

● Fresh okra contains a variety of the B vitamins as well as generous amounts of vitamin C, soluble fiber, and the carotenoids lutein and zeaxanthin.

Eggplant

SATURATED FAT g	PROTEIN g	CARBOHYDRATE g	FIBER g	SUGARS g	GI
tr	1	75	4.8	69	NA
tr	2	6	2.5	1.3	NA
tr	0	0.5	0.5	0	NA
tr	2	6	2	1.9	NA
tr	1	7	2.4	3.2	NA
tr	1	6	1.4	3.4	NA
.5	2	13	1.7	NA	NA

ONIONS, LEEKS, AND GARLIC

● ● ●

LOW IN CALORIES.
HIGH IN ANTIOXIDANTS

Not particularly high in vitamins or minerals, members of the allium family are high in flavor and in phytochemicals.

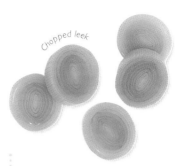

Chopped leek

Leeks

WHAT'S IN IT?

Scallions, sometimes called spring onions, are sold with their green tops attached. Don't discard them—they contain beta carotene.

TIP

● Sweet onions are actually slightly lower in sugars than regular yellow storage onions. They also contain fewer of the sulfur compounds that make onions so pungent, which results in their milder flavor.

STYLE 1 medium	CALORIES	CHOLESTEROL mg	SODIUM mg	TOTAL FAT g
Onion, cooked	41	0	3	0.2
Onion, raw	42	0	3	0.2
Shallot (1 tbsp)	7	0	1	tr
Garlic	4	0	0.5	tr
Leek	38	0	12	0.2
Scallion, top and bulb	8	9	4	tr

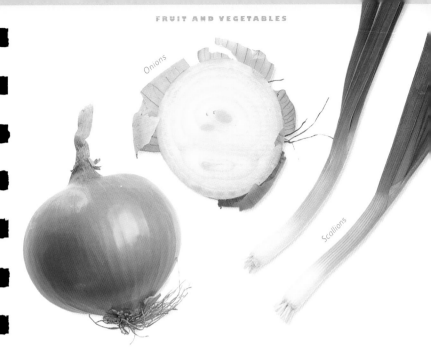

Onions

Scallions

WHAT'S THE BEST?

● Sulfur compounds. Onions contain diallyl sulfide, which is thought to neutralize cancer-causing agents. Garlic contains more than 100 sulfur compounds. Allicin, which gives garlic its aroma and flavor, forms when garlic is exposed to oxygen and takes about 10 minutes to develop. Heating garlic right after chopping or crushing it prevents allicin from forming, but once it has formed, heat won't destroy it.

WHAT'S NOT SO GOOD?

● Sulfur compounds—in your eyes and on your breath. Lessen tears by holding onions under running water as you peel them. To sweeten breath, chew fresh parsley or mint leaves.

Garlic

SATURATED FAT g	PROTEIN g	CARBOHYDRATE g	FIBER g	SUGARS g	GI
tr	1	10	1.3	9	NA
tr	1	9	2	6	NA
tr	0.3	2	NA	NA	NA
tr	0.2	1	0.1	tr	NA
tr	1	9	1.2	NA	NA
tr	0.5	2	0.7	0.8	NA

SALAD VEGETABLES

● ● ●

VERY LOW IN CALORIES

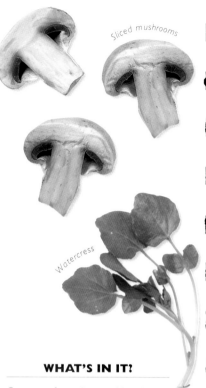

Sliced mushrooms

Watercress

Make dark leafy greens the focus of your salad bowl to minimize calories and maximize vitamins.

TIP

● Don't forget herbs! Basil, mint, and parsley add flavor and nutrients to salads.

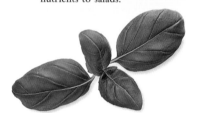

WHAT'S IN IT?

One cup of romaine provides about twice the calcium, phosphorus, iron, and potassium of iceberg; almost eight times the vitamin A; and about six times the vitamin C.

STYLE 1 cup shredded	CALORIES	CHOLESTEROL mg	SODIUM mg	TOTAL FAT g
Romaine	8	0	4	0.1
Arugula	5	0	5	0.1
Iceberg	6	0	5	tr
Watercress	4	0	14	tr
Spinach	7	0	24	0.1
Endive (½ cup)	4	0	6	tr
Additions to salad not found elsewhere:				
Mushrooms, sliced	18	0	3	0.2
Bean sprouts	16	0	3	0.1

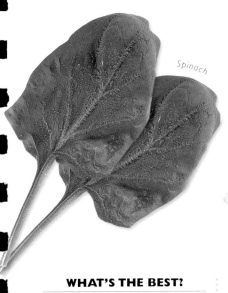

Spinach

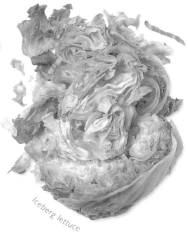

Iceberg lettuce

WHAT'S THE BEST?

● Spinach. By weight, it supplies almost as much beta carotene as pumpkin! Its chlorophyll hides the orange pigment.

● Cleaned greens. Plastic bags and boxes of greens make it easy to enjoy a variety of salad greens. Don't forget to give the greens a quick rinse or to pick through the leaves and remove any that are past their prime.

WHAT'S NOT SO GOOD?

● Bottled dressings. Instead, combine 3 parts olive oil and 1 part red wine or balsamic vinegar; add minced garlic, Dijon mustard, or chopped herbs.

● Paler greens. Iceberg and endive lack the vitamins and antioxidants of their deeper, darker counterparts.

SATURATED FAT g	PROTEIN g	CARBOHYDRATE g	FIBER g	SUGARS g	GI
tr	0.9	1.4	0.9	0.6	L
tr	0.5	1	0.3	0.4	L
tr	0.4	1	0.5	1	L
tr	0.8	0.5	0.6	tr	L
tr	0.9	1	0.8	0.2	L
tr	0.3	1	0.8	0.3	L
tr	2	3	0.8	1.3	L
0	2	3	0.9	1.1	L

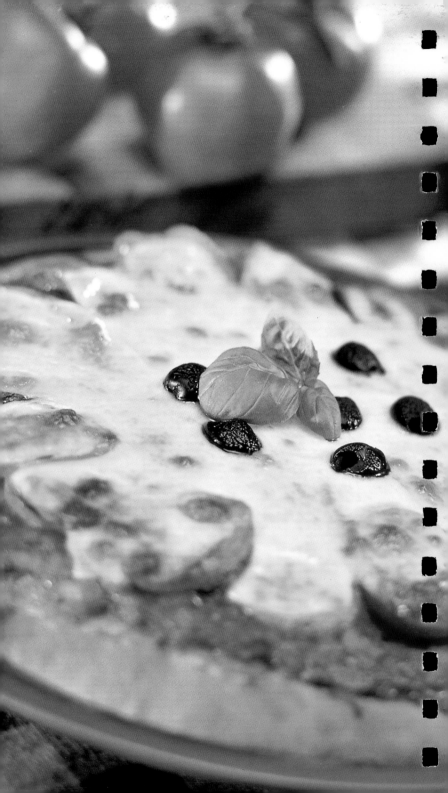

FAST FOOD AND DRINKS

Fast-food restaurants and snack and candy manufacturers are quick to tell you that their products can be part of a healthful diet. They're not so speedy, though, with practical tips—a single meal of a super burger, jumbo fries, mega soda, and fried pie can easily surpass a person's daily requirements for calories, fat, sugar, and sodium yet not come close to meeting the recommended amounts for vitamins and minerals.

The key is limits. Fast food, candy, and other snacks should be infrequent supplements to your diet, not its foundation. On the occasions you do indulge, keep portion sizes in mind. If you've got a craving for fries, get a small burger or a salad to go with it. Want some chocolate? Better to have one small, perfectly rich piece than a huge bar of so-so stuff. If you're too busy to cook, vary your diet—get takeout sushi, or a slice and a salad at a pizza parlor.

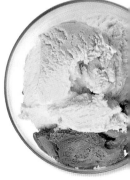

McDONALD'S

●

CHOOSE VERY CAREFULLY

*I*s it possible to eat healthfully at McDonald's? Yes, but it isn't easy.

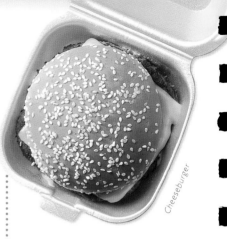

Cheeseburger

WHAT'S IN IT?

Two all-beef patties, special sauce, lettuce, cheese, pickles, onions, a sesame seed bun—that's 580 calories worth of food, with 33g fat and 47g carbs.

STYLE 1 serving	CALORIES	CHOLESTEROL mg	SODIUM mg	TOTAL FAT g
Hamburger	280	30	560	10
Cheeseburger	330	45	800	14
Big Mac	580	85	1050	33
Quarter Pounder	420	95	1250	21
Double Q.P. w/Cheese	760	165	1450	48
Small fries	210	0	135	10
Medium fries	450	0	290	22
Large fries	540	0	350	26
Super fries	610	0	390	29
Filet-O-Fish	470	50	730	26
Chicken McGrill	400	60	890	17
Crispy Chicken	500	50	1100	26
Chicken McNuggets (6 pieces)	310	50	680	20
Grilled Chicken Caesar Salad *	210	60	680	7
Grilled Chicken Caesar Salad **	400	80	1180	25
Crispy Chicken Caesar Salad *	310	50	890	16
Crispy Chicken Caesar Salad **	500	70	1390	34
Fruit 'n' Yogurt Parfait	380	15	240	5
Baked Apple Pie	260	0	200	13
Vanilla Triple Thick Shake (16 oz)	570	65	400	16

* w/o dressing ** w/dressing

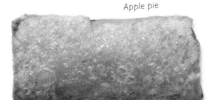

Apple pie

WHAT'S THE BEST?

● Smaller portions, always. Yes, the larger sizes give you more value if you're looking for quantity. But what if you're looking for health?

● If you're looking for a nutritional bargain, choose a salad, preferably one without the word "crispy" in the title. That's not-so-secret code for breaded or fried.

WHAT'S NOT SO GOOD?

● Do the math. Select what you usually order below, then turn to the the soda section (pages 196–197) and add up the numbers for your usual meal. Remember that the average woman needs 1,700–2,000 calories a day, the typical man 2000–2,700 calories, and that nutritionists recommend limiting sodium to 2,400mg per day.

SATURATED FAT g	PROTEIN g	CARBOHYDRATE g	FIBER g	SUGARS g	GI
4	12	35	2	7	NA
6	15	35	2	7	NA
11	24	47	3	7	NA
8	23	36	2	8	NA
20	46	38	2	9	NA
1.5	3	26	2	0	NA
4	6	57	5	0	NA
4.5	8	68	6	0	NA
5	9	77	7	0	NA
5	15	45	1	5	NA
3	25	37	2	6	NA
4.5	22	46	2	6	NA
4	15	18	2	0	NA
3.5	26	11	3	3	NA
7	28	15	3	5	NA
4.5	23	20	3	4	NA
8	25	24	3	6	NA
2	10	76	2	49	NA
3.5	3	34	<1	13	NA
11	14	89	0	76	NA

149

BURGER KING

●

CHOOSE VERY CAREFULLY

*F*ire-grilled burgers must be good for you. Right? Not necessarily. Don't forget to take into account how big that burger is, the fat content of the meat it's made of, as well as what you put on it.

A BK Veggie burger is somewhat more healthful, but it might not be vegetarian.

TIP

● Unlike some restaurants that limit kids' meals to those under age 12, fast-food restaurants sell kids' meals to anyone. Order one to keep your portion sizes in line.

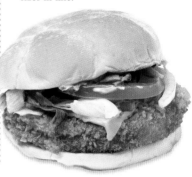

STYLE 1 serving	CALORIES	CHOLESTEROL mg	SODIUM mg	TOTAL FAT g
Hamburger	310	40	580	13
Double Cheeseburger	540	100	1050	31
Whopper	710	85	980	43
Whopper Jr. w/Cheese	440	55	790	26
Small fries	230	0	410	11
Medium fries	360	0	640	18
Large fries	500	0	880	25
King size fries	600	0	1070	30
BK Veggie (no mayo)	340	0	950	10
Original Chicken Sandwich	565	65	1270	28
Chicken Whopper Sandwich	580	75	1370	26
Baked Potato w/Chives	260	0	20	0
Chili	216	0	1040	8
Chicken Caesar Salad (w/o dressing or croutons)	225	65	1040	7
Chicken Caesar Salad (w/dressing)	360	75	1385	20
Chicken Caesar Salad (w/dressing and croutons)	450	75	1685	23

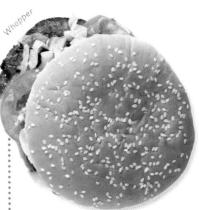

Whopper

WHAT'S IN IT?

Burger King's Web site makes no promises that its BK Veggie burger conforms to a vegan or vegetarian, diet. The patty itself may be meat-free but it's cooked on the same grill as the beef burgers.

WHAT'S THE BEST?

● Salads are a good option. Remember that if you choose a nonfat or reduced-fat salad dressing, it's probably high in carbohydrate.

● Infrequent occasions. If you zip through the drive-thru on a regular basis, you're not doing yourself any favors.

WHAT'S NOT SO GOOD?

● Expanding portion sizes. Fifty years ago, a Burger King hamburger weighed about 1/4 pound, including bun and pickles. Now, a regular hamburger weighs a little over 1/4 pound, and a Whopper? A whopping 10 1/4 oz.

SATURATED FAT g	PROTEIN g	CARBOHYDRATE g	FIBER g	SUGARS g	GI
5	17	31	2	6	NA
15	32	32	2	6	NA
13	31	52	4	11	NA
9	19	32	2	6	NA
3	3	29	2	0	NA
5	4	46	4	1	NA
7	6	63	5	1	NA
8	7	76	6	1	NA
1.5	14	47	4	8	NA
6	25	52	3	5	NA
5	39	48	4	7	NA
0	6	61	6	5	NA
3	25	17	5	5	NA
3	36	5	3	3	NA
5	37	9	3	5	NA
5.5	39	23	3	6	NA

KFC

● ●

SOME HEALTHFUL OPTIONS

A few years ago, Kentucky Fried Chicken became KFC. Even though "fried" is no longer part of the name, frying is still the primary cooking method.

Original recipe

TIP

● You'll reduce fat, calories, carbohydrate, and sodium by removing the skin and highly seasoned breading. Or just choose roast chicken and save yourself the extra step.

WHAT'S IN IT?

Removing the skin won't reduce the cholesterol significantly. That's because a lot of the cholesterol is in the lean tissue, not skin.

STYLE 1 serving	CALORIES	CHOLESTEROL mg	SODIUM mg	TOTAL FAT g
Original Recipe Breast	370	145	1145	19
Extra Crispy Breast	470	135	1230	28
Hot & Spicy Breast	179	130	1450	27
Triple Crunch Sandwich w/sauce	490	70	710	29
Tender Roast Sandwich w/sauce	350	75	880	15
Tender Roast Sandwich w/o sauce	270	65	690	5
Chunky Chicken Pot Pie	770	70	2160	42
Hot Wings	471	150	1230	33
Mashed Potatoes w/gravy	120	<1	440	6
Green Beans	45	5	730	1.5
Mean Greens	70	10	650	3
Pecan Pie Slice	490	65	510	23
Little Bucket Parfait-Strawberry Shortcake	200	19	220	7

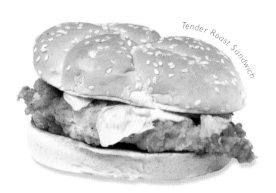

Tender Roast Sandwich

WHAT'S THE BEST?

● Veggies. KFC is one of the few fast-food restaurants to offer vegetables other than fried potatoes. Go for the greens or the beans.

● Tender Roast Sandwich. If you're watching your carb intake, eat it with a knife and fork (or ask for extra lettuce and use the leaves as a wrap).

WHAT'S NOT SO GOOD?

● Crispy, crunchy, and barbecue. These terms signify high carbohydrate, either from refined flours or sugar, and high fat—usually trans fat.

● Pot pie. Sounds healthful? OK, it provides 80 percent of the Daily Value for vitamin A, but it supplies 90 percent of the Daily Value for sodium, too.

SATURATED FAT g	PROTEIN g	CARBOHYDRATE g	FIBER g	SUGARS g	GI
6	40	11	0	0	NA
8	34	19	0	0	NA
8	33	20	0	0	NA
6	28	39	2	0	NA
3	32	26	1	1	NA
1.5	31	23	1	<1	NA
13	29	69	5	8	NA
8	27	18	2	0	NA
1	1	17	2	0	NA
0.5	1	7	3	3	NA
1	4	11	5	1	NA
5	5	66	2	31	NA
6	1	33	1	26	NA

TACO BELL

●

CHOOSE VERY CAREFULLY

*T*aco Bell's offerings tend to be lower in cholesterol and higher in fiber than most fast-food options. However, they're still quite high in total fat and sodium, so you'll want to choose your meal carefully.

TIP

● If you're limiting fat, opt for a burrito or something wrapped in a flour tortilla. If you're limiting carbs, choose a corn tortilla. Corn tortillas are lower in carbohydrates, but because they're usually fried, they're higher in fat.

WHAT'S IN IT?

Cheese supplies calcium and protein, and beans supply fiber as well as protein. Both are higher in carbohydrate than meat. Steer clear of the crispy taco shells, which are high in fat and carbohydrate.

Don't remove the lettuce from your taco, particularly if it's vitamin-rich romaine.

STYLE 1 serving	CALORIES	CHOLESTEROL mg	SODIUM mg	TOTAL FAT g
Taco Supreme	220	40	360	14
Grilled Steak Soft Taco	280	30	650	17
Double Decker Taco	340	25	800	14
Gordita Baja, Chicken	320	40	690	15
Chalupa Supreme, Beef	390	40	600	24
Bean Burrito	370	10	1200	10
Grilled Stuft Burrito, Steak	680	55	1940	28
Taco Salad w/Shell	790	65	1670	42
Taco Salad w/o Shell	420	65	1400	21
Chicken Quesadilla	540	80	1380	30
Nachos	320	<5	530	19
Pintos 'n Cheese	180	15	700	7

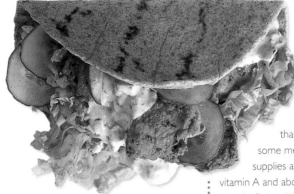

 You might find romaine lettuce, rather than iceberg, offered on some menu items. Romaine supplies almost 8 times more vitamin A and about 6 times more vitamin C than iceberg—ask for it on your meal.

Choose a flour tortilla over corn tortilla—these will contain less fat. Ordering vegetables will help boost the nutritional content, too.

WHAT'S NOT SO GOOD?

● Salads. Even the smaller Express Taco Salad comes with chips, increasing its fat and carb content. The Taco Salad in the shell is higher in saturated fat, calories, carbs and sodium than a Big Mac or a Whopper (but it does have 1g less total fat than a Whopper).

WHAT'S THE BEST?

● Order extra veggies on your meal in order to boost vitamins and nutrients. Green Sauce, Red Sauce, and Salsa can add flavor without doing much damage.

SATURATED FAT g	PROTEIN g	CARBOHYDRATE g	FIBER g	SUGARS g	GI
7	9	14	3	2	NA
4.5	12	21	1	3	NA
5	15	39	6	3	NA
3.5	17	29	7	2	NA
10	14	31	5	3	NA
3.5	14	55	8	4	NA
8	31	76	6	6	NA
15	31	73	13	10	NA
11	24	33	11	9	NA
13	28	40	2	4	NA
4.5	5	33	2	3	NA
3.5	10	20	6	1	NA

PIZZA

● ●

CAN BE HEART-HEALTHY

*G*o for the thinnest crust, the least cheese, and the most vegetables for the healthiest pizza.

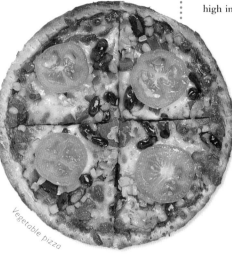

Vegetable pizza

WHAT'S IN IT?

Tomato sauce is high in lycopene, a cancer-fighting carotenoid. Cheese provides good amounts of calcium and protein, and some pizza parlors offer whole-wheat crusts.

STYLE 1 slice	CALORIES	CHOLESTEROL mg	SODIUM mg	TOTAL FAT g
Pizza Hut				
Pepperoni, Thin 'N Crispy	190	15	610	9
Cheese, Thin 'N Crispy	200	10	590	0
Meat Lover's Stuffed Crust	470	50	1430	25
Beef, Personal Pan	710	45	1580	35
Veggie Lover's, Hand Tossed	250	5	580	8
Domino's (1 slice of 12-inch pie)				
Cheese, Hand Tossed	187	11	388	5.5
Vegi Feast, Hand Tossed	220	17	494	7.9
Pepperoni Feast	267	29	674	12.3
ExtravaganZZa Feast	288	32	756	13.4

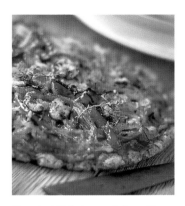

For a healthful pizza, ask for a thin, whole-wheat crust.

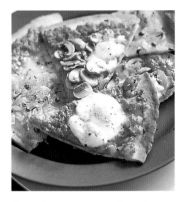

Extra cheese means extra fat and extra sodium. Don't ask for it!

WHAT'S THE BEST?

● Extra napkins. Pizza—pepperoni in particular—can have a lot of grease on top. Blot off as much as you can.

● Veggie pizzas. They're an easy way to add vegetables to your diet.

● Homemade. Keep pizza dough on hand and make your own in less time than it takes to have a pie delivered.

WHAT'S NOT SO GOOD?

● Veggie pizzas. They're not always that high in nutritious vegetables. Go light on the mushrooms and onions and opt for more broccoli, spinach, or tomatoes.

● Extra cheese and most meat toppings. Sausage and pepperoni tend to be very high in sodium.

SATURATED FAT g	PROTEIN g	CARBOHYDRATE g	FIBER g	SUGARS g	GI
4	9	21	2	1	NA
5	10	22	2	1	NA
11	16	40	3	2	NA
14	31	71	6	<2	NA
3	9	29	2	2	NA
2.4	8	27	1.5	2.3	NA
3.6	10	27	1.9	2.5	NA
5.5	12	28	1.6	2.5	NA
5.8	13	29	2	2.7	NA

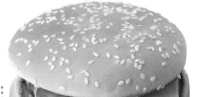

Classic Single with Cheese

WENDY'S

● ●

SOME HEALTHFUL OPTIONS

W*endy's offers several options beyond burgers. Their salads have earned a reputation for high flavor and freshness.*

TIP

● For a fresher meal, make a special order. Ask for a sandwich with no ketchup or mustard, for example, and then add your own at the table.

WHAT'S IN IT?

The only difference between a Jr. Hamburger and a Kids' Meal Hamburger is that the former includes onions. A Jr. Cheeseburger Deluxe and a Classic Single with Cheese are identical except for the size of the hamburger patty.

STYLE 1 serving	CALORIES	CHOLESTEROL mg	SODIUM mg	TOTAL FAT g
Classic Single w/everything	410	70	890	19
Big Bacon Classic	570	100	1460	29
Kids' Meal Hamburger	270	30	600	9
Grilled Chicken Sandwich	300	55	740	7
Spicy Chicken Sandwich	430	60	1240	15
Caesar Side Salad w/o dressing	70	15	250	4
Caesar Side Salad w/dressing	220	35	490	20
Caesar Side Salad w/dressing and garlic croutons	290	35	610	22.5
Spring Mix Salad	180	30	230	11
Honey Roasted Pecans	130	0	65	13
House Vinaigrette	190	9	750	18
Broccoli & Cheese Stuffed Baked Potato	480	5	510	14
Chili, large	300	50	1310	9
Chicken Nuggets (5)	220	35	480	14
Frosty, medium	440	50	260	11
Fries (see page 162)				

WHAT'S THE BEST?

● Salads. Wendy's Spring Mix Salad is heavy on the vegetables, and the Mandarin Chicken Salad with Roasted Almonds is a good choice if you skip the optional Crispy Rice Noodles. If you order the Caesar Side Salad, pass on the croutons, which contain trans fats.

● Grilled chicken. Breaded chicken, whether in nugget form or "fillets," is sometimes made from chicken scraps that are pressed together and cut to size. Such manipulation is harder to fake with a grilled chicken breast.

WHAT'S NOT SO GOOD?

● Doubles and Triples. Each additional patty adds 200 calories, 14g fat, 19g protein, 290mg sodium, and 65mg cholesterol. Keep portions smaller with the Classic Single, or with a Jr. Hamburger.

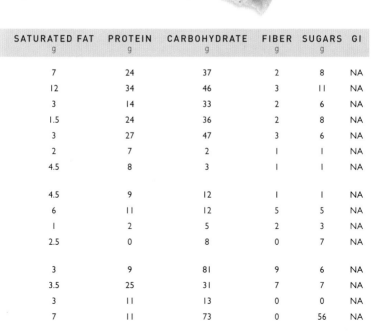

Chicken nuggets

SATURATED FAT g	PROTEIN g	CARBOHYDRATE g	FIBER g	SUGARS g	GI
7	24	37	2	8	NA
12	34	46	3	11	NA
3	14	33	2	6	NA
1.5	24	36	2	8	NA
3	27	47	3	6	NA
2	7	2	1	1	NA
4.5	8	3	1	1	NA
4.5	9	12	1	1	NA
6	11	12	5	5	NA
1	2	5	2	3	NA
2.5	0	8	0	7	NA
3	9	81	9	6	NA
3.5	25	31	7	7	NA
3	11	13	0	0	NA
7	11	73	0	56	NA

SUBWAY

CAN BE HEART-HEALTHY

S ubway was in the news when a young man lost more than 200 pounds on a diet that included two Subway sandwiches a day.

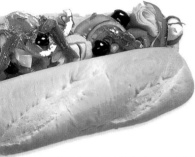

WHAT'S IN IT?

Subway's bread choices aren't as healthful as you might think. The Wheat Bread is made primarily with enriched white flour, and the Honey Oat Bread is simply the Wheat Bread with a sweet topping.

TIP

● Opt for vinegar and olive oil on your sandwich, not mayo. You won't save calories, but the fat is monounsaturated.

Add lots of flavor—and beneficial fats—to your sandwich with a sprinkling of pitted olives.

STYLE 1 serving	CALORIES	CHOLESTEROL mg	SODIUM mg	TOTAL FAT g
6-inch Roast Beef	290	20	910	5
Roast Beef on Deli Round	220	15	660	4.5
6-inch Meatball	540	45	1300	26
Tuna on Deli Round	330	25	830	16
Dijon Horseradish Melt	470	40	1620	21
Double Meat Chicken	410	90	1500	8
Turkey Breast & Ham Salad, without dressing	120	25	1030	3
Italian BMT Salad, without Dressing	280	55	1590	19
Roasted Chicken Noodle Soup	90	20	1180	4
Cream of Potato with Broccoli	210	20	970	12
Minestrone	70	10	1030	1
Apple Pie	245	0	290	10
Berry Lishus Fruizle Express (small)	110	0	30	0

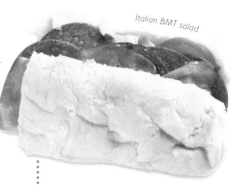

Italian BMT salad

WHAT'S THE BEST?

● Subway features ten sandwiches with 6g of fat or less. Those on Deli Rounds are lower in calories, carbohydrate, and sodium than those on 6-inch breads.

● Salads and soups provide nutritious alternatives to typical fast-food sides like fries. Studies have shown that if you eat soup before your entrée, you'll consume fewer total calories at the meal. If your favorite sandwich is one of the higher-fat ones or you're also ordering fries, choose a lower-fat soup like Roasted Chicken Noodle or Minestrone.

WHAT'S NOT SO GOOD?

● Stray from Subway's lean options and you're in the same nutrient desert as other fast-food restaurants.

● Steer clear of cured meats and cold cuts such as salami, bologna, and ham, which are high in nitrates and sodium. The tuna salad isn't the most nutritious choice, either.

SATURATED FAT g	PROTEIN g	CARBOHYDRATE g	FIBER g	SUGARS g	GI
2	19	46	4	7	NA
1.5	13	35	3	4	NA
11	23	53	5	8	NA
4.5	13	36	3	3	NA
7	26	48	4	6	NA
3	37	50	5	9	NA
0.5	12	11	3	3	NA
8	16	12	3	4	NA
1	7	7	1	1	NA
4	5	20	4	3	NA
0	3	11	2	2	NA
2	0	37	1	25	NA
0	1	28	1	27	NA

FRENCH FRIES

●

NOT HEART-HEALTHY.
HIGH IN FAT AND CARBS

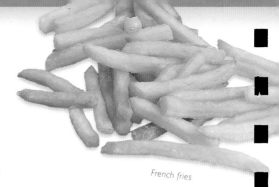

French fries

Potatoes are high in vitamin C and low in fat, but fry them in lots of oil and they lose a significant amount of vitamins and the amount of fat skyrockets. Add salt and the nutritional value plummets further.

WHAT'S IN IT?

Commercial fries, whether from supermarkets or restaurants can be made from reconstituted potato scraps and are high in trans fats. Cooking oils break down when heated, so restaurant fries may also contain potentially harmful chemicals.

STYLE medium serving	CALORIES	CHOLESTEROL mg	SODIUM mg	TOTAL FAT g
Arby's Curly Fries	400	0	990	20
Arby's Homestyle Fries	370	0	710	16
KFC Potato Wedges	376	4	1323	15
McDonald's				
Small fries	210	0	135	10
Medium fries	450	0	290	22
Large fries	540	0	350	26
Super fries	610	0	390	29
Wendy's				
Kid's Meal fries	250	0	220	11
Medium fries	390	0	340	17
Biggie fries	440	0	380	19
Great Biggie fries	530	0	450	23
Burger King				
Small fries	230	0	410	11
Medium fries	360	0	640	18
Large fries	500	0	880	25
King size fries	600	0	1070	30
Supermarket fries (3-oz serving)				
Shoestring	150	0	29	6
Steak fries	110	0	20	3

WHAT'S THE BEST?

● Homemade and oven-baked. You'll be hard pressed to find nutritious fries in a fast-food restaurant. Most are fried in partially hydrogenated oils and are loaded with trans fats. Cut up scrubbed potatoes (leave the peel on), drizzle them with canola oil, and bake them for a healthful alternative.

WHAT'S NOT SO GOOD?

● Salt. If you're sensitive to sodium, try sprinkling fries with a salt-free seasoning blend.

● Skinny fries. It's a lot easier to grab a bunch of shoestring-cut fries than a handful of steak fries, so it's a lot easier to eat more shoestrings.

● Big portions. Resist the urge to go with the jumbo fries. Medium, or better yet small, is a better bet.

TIP

● Thicker and larger fries can be lower in fat and salt than thin varieties because ounce for ounce they have less surface area.

SATURATED FAT g	PROTEIN g	CARBOHYDRATE g	FIBER g	SUGARS g	GI
5	5	50	3	NA	NA
4	4	53	4	NA	NA
4.2	6.2	53	4.5	<1	NA
1.5	3	26	2	0	NA
4	6	57	5	0	NA
4.5	8	68	6	0	NA
5	9	77	7	0	NA
2	3	36	4	0	NA
3	4	56	6	0	NA
3.5	5	63	7	0	NA
4.5	6	75	8	1	NA
3	3	29	2	0	NA
5	4	46	4	1	NA
7	6	63	5	1	NA
8	7	76	6	1	NA
0.5	2	22	2	0	NA
0.5	2	19	1	0	NA

FAST-FOOD BREAKFAST OPTIONS

●

NOT HEALTHFUL

While fast-food lunch and dinner options are redeemed—slightly—by vegetables, fast-food breakfasts are not.

WHAT'S IN IT?

Healthful fast-food breakfast options are few and far between. Most are full of fat, carbs, and sodium. Muffins, for instance, are rarely as healthful as you might think—in fact, some can be richer than cake.

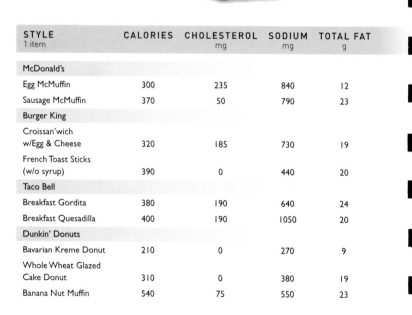

Egg McMuffin

STYLE 1 item	CALORIES	CHOLESTEROL mg	SODIUM mg	TOTAL FAT g
McDonald's				
Egg McMuffin	300	235	840	12
Sausage McMuffin	370	50	790	23
Burger King				
Croissan'wich w/Egg & Cheese	320	185	730	19
French Toast Sticks (w/o syrup)	390	0	440	20
Taco Bell				
Breakfast Gordita	380	190	640	24
Breakfast Quesadilla	400	190	1050	20
Dunkin' Donuts				
Bavarian Kreme Donut	210	0	270	9
Whole Wheat Glazed Cake Donut	310	0	380	19
Banana Nut Muffin	540	75	550	23

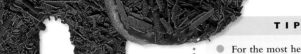
Doughnuts

WHAT'S THE BEST?

● Pickings are slim. If you're looking for acceptable nutrition, go with eggs—just be aware that most fast-food restaurants start with reconstituted frozen egg "patties" that are reheated beforehand.

● Unless 100 percent whole-wheat is an option, skip the bread. Muffins, croissants, doughnuts, and pastries contain trans fats.

TIP

● For the most healthful breakfasts, skip the fast-food restaurants entirely. If you're too pressed for time to eat at home, stop at a deli or convenience store, where you may be able to pick up a cup of yogurt or a piece of fruit.

WHAT'S NOT SO GOOD?

● Don't be fooled. Yes, fruit and whole wheat are full of beneficial nutrients, but when these words are used to describe a doughnut they're no longer healthful.

● Meats like bacon and sausage are high in nitrates and sodium.

SATURATED FAT g	PROTEIN g	CARBOHYDRATE g	FIBER g	SUGARS g	GI
5	18	29	2	3	NA
9	14	28	2	2	NA
7	12	24	<1	3	NA
4.5	6	30	2	11	NA
7	14	28	2	6	NA
9	17	38	3	3	NA
2	3	30	1	9	NA
4	4	32	2	14	NA
6	10	73	3	35	NA

FAST-FOOD FISH

●

CHOOSE VERY CAREFULLY

Although fish is low in fat, free of carbohydrate, and can be high in heart-healthy omega-3 essential fatty acids, you'd never know if from a fast-food menu.

TIP

● Scan the menu to see if there are any grilled or broiled options. If not, you're better off removing the breaded coating. It protects the fish from absorbing a lot of fat.

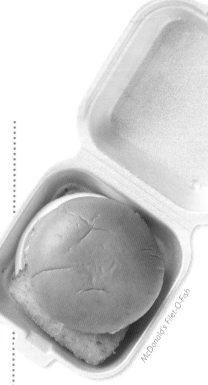

McDonald's Filet-O-Fish

WHAT'S IN IT?

Most fast-food fish is breaded or batter-dipped, then deep-fried. It's high in trans fats and refined flour, and rivals burgers and cheeseburgers in fat, cholesterol, and carb content.

STYLE 1 serving, unless noted	CALORIES	CHOLESTEROL mg	SODIUM mg	TOTAL FAT g
Fried fish (1 fillet)	211	31	484	11.2
Fish sandwich w/tartar sauce	431	55	615	22.8
Fried clams (¾ cup)	451	87	834	26.4
Fried shrimp (6–8)	454	200	1446	24.9
Fried oysters (6)	368	108	677	17.9
McDonald's Filet-O-Fish	470	50	730	26

WHAT'S THE BEST?

● If salmon is on the menu—more likely at someplace like Red Lobster than Long John Silver—it's one of the better choices. Although salmon is fattier than some other fish, it's also an excellent source of omega-3s.

● Skip the white bread. Whole-wheat, whole-grain, and even rye bread will give you a boost of nutrients and fiber.

WHAT'S NOT SO GOOD?

● Where to start? There's so little about deep-fried foods that's good, even a good-for-you food like fish. If you get cravings for fried clams, resist the urge to indulge them on anything resembling a frequent basis.

Fried fish and French fries can be a double dose of trans fats. Better to choose one or the other, not both.

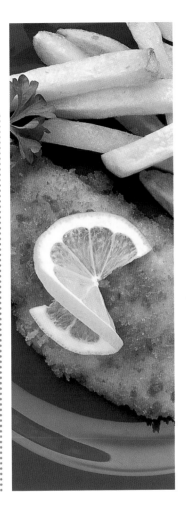

SATURATED FAT g	PROTEIN g	CARBOHYDRATE g	FIBER g	SUGARS g	GI
2.6	13	15	0.5	NA	NA
5.2	17	41	0	NA	NA
6.6	13	39	0	NA	NA
5.4	19	40	0	NA	NA
4.6	13	40	0	NA	NA
5	15	45	1	5	NA

SANDWICHES AND SUBS

● ●

SOME HEALTHFUL OPTIONS

*I*f you're not worried about sodium, saturated and trans fats, nitrates from cured meats, or carbohydrates, you'll find some healthful options in sandwiches.

TIP

● Most delis overstuff sandwiches. See if you can have yours made with a smaller amount of meat, or save the extras for another meal. Because most deli and cold cuts are very high in sodium, opt for a green salad, heavy on the vegetables, as a side dish rather than a bag of chips.

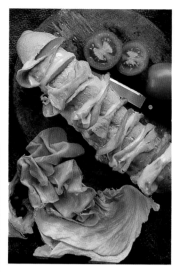

Sandwiches can be a healthful option, but don't let the deli stuff it with too much meat and cheese.

WHAT'S IN IT?

One fast-food deli offers a large corned beef sandwich with more than 1,100 calories—more than half of what the typical woman needs in a day—and almost 4,800mg sodium —about double the recommended daily amount.

STYLE 1 serving	CALORIES	CHOLESTEROL mg	SODIUM mg	TOTAL FAT g
Sub with cold cuts	456	36	1651	18.6
Turkey half sub w/mayo	561	102	2021	34.8
Turkey half sub w/o mayo	325	72	2021	8.5
Roast beef sub	410	73	845	13
Tuna salad sub	584	49	1293	28
Ham and cheese	352	58	771	15.5
Steak sandwich	459	73	798	14
Hot dog	242	44	670	14.5
Chili dog	296	51	480	13.4

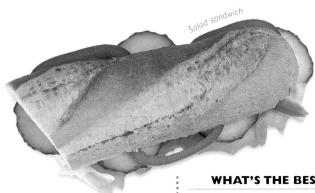

Salad sandwich

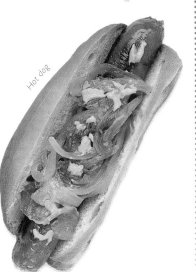

Hot dog

WHAT'S THE BEST?

● Small portions. The smallest version of the corned beef sandwich, mentioned opposite in "What's in it?," provides a manageable 400 calories and about 1600mg sodium.

WHAT'S NOT SO GOOD?

● Club sandwiches. An extra slice of bread and the extra layer of sandwich fillings add a lot more food than most people need.

● Grilled sandwiches. Not "grilled" as in "cooked on an open flame with lots of smoky flavor"; most sandwiches are grilled as in "slathered with butter and fried on a grill."

SATURATED FAT g	PROTEIN g	CARBOHYDRATE g	FIBER g	SUGARS g	GI
6.8	22	51	NA	NA	NA
12	32	30	NA	NA	NA
3	32	30	NA	NA	NA
7	27	44	NA	NA	NA
5.3	30	55	NA	NA	NA
6.4	21	33	NA	NA	NA
3.8	20	52	NA	NA	NA
5.1	10	18	NA	NA	NA
4.9	14	21	NA	NA	NA

CHIPS, PRETZELS, AND SAVORY SNACKS

●

CAN BE HIGH IN TRANS FATS

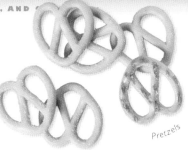
Pretzels

*D*on't be impressed by labels trumpeting "cholesterol-free!" The only foods that have cholesterol are those from animals— meat, dairy, and eggs—not from vegetables or grains.

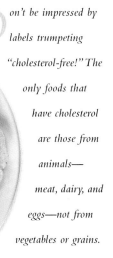
Plain chips

WHAT'S IN IT?

Labels for plain potato chips can list "potatoes, oil, and salt." Some flavored chips have ingredients lists that seem to run on for paragraphs.

TIPS

● Most snack food bags are full of air—not to delude consumers into thinking that they're getting a lot of chips, but to provide a cushion to keep chips from breaking.

● Look on the Nutrition Facts label to see how many chips are in a serving. Count out the whole chips, then compare them to your usual handful.

STYLE 1 serving	CALORIES	CHOLESTEROL mg	SODIUM mg	TOTAL FAT g
Plain chips	150	0	180	10
Barbecue chips	150	0	200	10
Baked chips	110	0	150	1.5
Fat-free chips	75	0	200	0
Corn chips	160	0	170	10
Cheesy puffs	160	0	370	10
Nacho tortilla chips	140	0	200	7
Pretzels twists, mini	120	0	420	1
Popcorn, air-popped	108	0	1	1.2
Popcorn, oil-popped	142	0	251	8
Rice and corn puffs	140	0	130	6

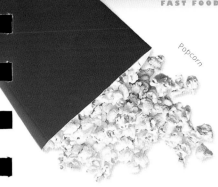

Popcorn

WHAT'S THE BEST?

● Some chip manufacturers are frying their chips in oils that haven't been hydrogenated. These chips and snacks may be free of trans fats. (It may be easier to find trans fat-free chips in natural foods stores.)

● Single-serving packages. Yes, you pay a premium for the extra packaging, but if chips are your weakness these can make it easier to be aware of how much you're eating.

● Portion awareness. One ounce of oil-popped popcorn is about 2½ cups. Some movie theater buckets can equal 30 (yes, thirty) cups.

WHAT'S NOT SO GOOD?

● Shifting portion sizes. The information below is for 1 oz. That's the amount given on large bags as a serving. Watch for 2–3-oz bags. You might eat the contents as a single serving, but the Nutrition Facts information is probably based on 1-oz servings.

● Baked and fat-free chips. Lower in calories (and some say in flavor), these can make it all to easy to give yourself license to eat in large portions.

● "Healthy" snacks. Just because it's made with organic ingredients or you find it in a natural foods store doesn't mean it's good for you. Check labels to be sure there are no trans fats.

SATURATED FAT g	PROTEIN g	CARBOHYDRATE g	FIBER g	SUGARS g	GI
3	2	15	1	0	NA
3	2	15	1	2	NA
0	2	23	2	2	NA
0	2	18	1	0	NA
1.5	2	15	1	<1	H
2.5	2	15	<1	<1	NA
1.5	2	17	1	2	NA
0	2	23	1	<1	NA
0.2	3	22	4.3	NA	L
1.4	3	16	2.8	NA	L
0.5	2	17	0	0	H

CRACKERS

●

NOT HEART-HEALTHY

Crackers run the gamut from savory to plain to sweet. Although few can be called healthful, some are fairly benign.

WHAT'S IN IT?

Most crackers are made with refined flours and partially hydrogenated fats. They're high in carbohydrate and fat, particularly trans fats, and sodium.

It may be made of whole-wheat flour, but a cracker may still be high in trans fats.

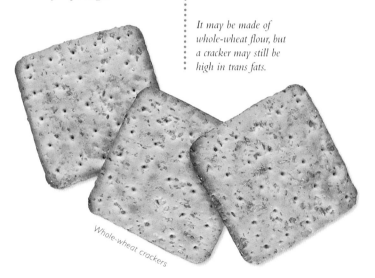

Whole-wheat crackers

STYLE 1 cracker	CALORIES	CHOLESTEROL mg	SODIUM mg	TOTAL FAT g
Saltine	13	0	39	0.4
Graham (2½-inch sq)	30	0	42	0.7
Matzo, plain	111	0	0.6	0.4
Melba toast, wheat	19	0	42	0.1
Rye crispbread	37	0	26	0.1
Round butter flavor	15	0	25	0.8
Small cheese crackers (1-oz single-serving bag)	141	3.6	279	7
Whole-wheat	18	0	26	0.7

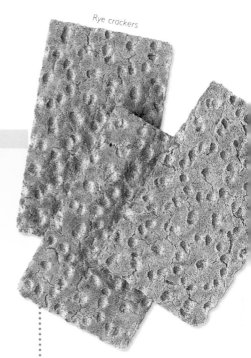

Rye crackers

WHAT'S THE BEST?

● Whole-grain crackers. Graham crackers contain whole-wheat flour. Crispbread or flat breads are often made with rye and other whole grains. Unlike most crackers, crispbreads are often fat-free.

WHAT'S NOT SO GOOD?

● Most commercial brands. Crackers and baked goods are almost always made with partially hydrogenated oils. These chemically modified fats raise cholesterol levels even more than saturated fats do.

SATURATED FAT g	PROTEIN g	CARBOHYDRATE g	FIBER g	SUGARS g	GI
tr	0.3	2	tr	NA	NA
0.1	0.5	5	0.2	1.3	NA
tr	3	23	0.8	NA	NA
tr	0.6	3.8	0.4	NA	H
tr	0.8	8	1.7	NA	M
tr	0.2	1.8	tr	NA	NA
2.6	3	16	0.7	NA	NA
0.1	0.4	2.7	0.4	NA	NA

DIPS

● ●

CAN BE HEART-HEALTHY

If your idea of dip is sour cream with some flavorings, accompanied by a good sturdy rippled potato chip, it's time to expand your horizons.

TIP

● Yogurt cheese is a good substitute for mayo and sour cream in dips. To make it, line a colander with paper towels or a cone-shaped coffee filter, then spoon in double the amount of yogurt that you need. Set over a bowl, then cover with plastic and refrigerate 5 hours. As the whey, or liquid, drains into the bowl the yogurt will thicken in consistency.

WHAT'S IN IT?

Sour cream-based dips are high in fat but very little else. Bean-, vegetable-, and cheese-based dips are high in protein and nutrients.

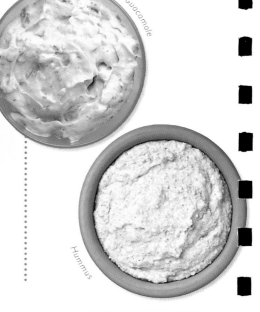

Guacamole

Hummus

STYLE 2 tablespoons	CALORIES	CHOLESTEROL mg	SODIUM mg	TOTAL FAT g
Hummus, homemade	51	0	73	2.5
Black bean dip	30	0	210	0
Cheddar cheese dip	60	5	330	4
Onion dip	50	<5	230	5
Guacamole	60	0	150	5
Salsa	9	0	139	tr

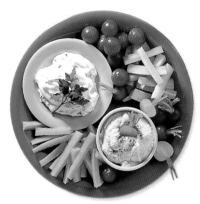

A dip made from yogurt
is a low-fat option.

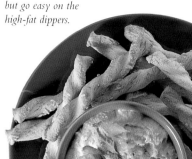

*Hummus is healthful,
but go easy on the
high-fat dippers.*

WHAT'S THE BEST?

● Guacamole. For a fast and delicious version, mix mashed avocado with your favorite chunky salsa. Use it as a sandwich spread or as a topping for grilled fish or meats.

● Hummus. High in fiber and protein, hummus and other bean dips are easy and inexpensive to make at home. Experiment with different beans and seasonings.

● Salsa. Most are tomato-based, which makes them a good source of the potent antioxidant lycopene.

WHAT'S NOT SO GOOD?

● Storebought dips. They're higher in additives and preservatives, and they rarely taste as good as homemade dips.

● Chips. Boost the nutrients in your nosh with vegetables—use bell pepper strips, kohlrabi rounds, broccoli florets, sticks of celery, or baby carrots as dippers.

SATURATED FAT g	PROTEIN g	CARBOHYDRATE g	FIBER g	SUGARS g	GI
0.4	1	6	1.5	NA	NA
0	2	6	2	<1	NA
1.5	1	3	0	<1	NA
2	1	2	<1	<1	NA
NA	1	3	2	NA	NA
tr	0.4	2	0.5	NA	NA

ICE CREAM, SORBET, AND SHERBET

●

MOST ARE HIGH IN SUGAR

*C*ool and refreshing, iced desserts can hit the spot on a hot summer night. While none can really be considered healthful, some are less harmful than others.

TIP

● Ice cream almost always includes cream as well as milk. Sherbet is typically made with a combination of milk and fruit juice. Sorbet never contains milk.

WHAT'S IN IT?

Super-premium ice creams, such as Haagen-Dazs, have less air whipped into them than premium and other varieties. As a result, they are denser in calories and other nutrients. If you go for quality over quantity, you may be satisfied with smaller amounts of these richer desserts.

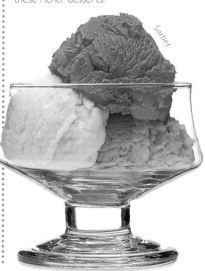

Sorbet

STYLE 1/2-cup serving	CALORIES	CHOLESTEROL mg	SODIUM mg	TOTAL FAT g
Haagen-Dazs Vanilla Swiss Almond ice cream	300	105	75	20
Haagen-Dazs Dulce de Leche ice cream	290	100	95	17
Premium, vanilla	145	32	58	7.9
Chocolate-covered ice cream bar (1 bar)	488	40	108	35.7
Orange sherbet	102	4	34	1.5
Haagen-Dazs Chocolate sorbet	120	0	70	0
French vanilla soft-serve	185	78	52	11.2

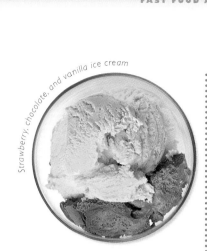

Strawberry, chocolate, and vanilla ice cream

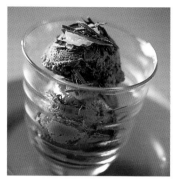

Chocolate ice cream

WHAT'S THE BEST?

● Ice creams for different dietary restrictions abound, though they can vary in quality from one brand to another. Try low-fat, sugar-free, or low-carb varieties—just don't use their lower numbers as an excuse to eat more.

● Look for high-calcium ice cream. It's not any lower in fat or sugar than regular ice cream, but additional milk powder adds a boost of this bone-building mineral.

WHAT'S NOT SO GOOD?

● Sundaes. Start adding toppings like fudge sauce, butterscotch sauce, whipped cream, sprinkles, and cherries and you'll easily add hundreds of calories, not to mention alarming amounts of fat and sugar. Even the nutritional benefits of a good-for-you topping like nuts won't help to redeem your dessert.

● Two or three scoops. Take the numbers below and double or triple them.

SATURATED FAT g	PROTEIN g	CARBOHYDRATE g	FIBER g	SUGARS g	GI
11	5	24	<1	21	M
10	5	28	0	28	NA
4.9	3	17	0.5	12.7	M
19.4	6	36	0	30.6	NA
0.9	0.8	22	0	18	NA
0	2	28	2	20	NA
6.4	4	19	0	NA	NA

PUDDING, MOUSSE, AND CUSTARD

●

CAN BE HIGH IN CALCIUM

For some, rich and creamy pudding and custard desserts are the ultimate comfort food. Look for recipes that are lower in sugar or fat, but be careful about substituting low-carb sweeteners or low-fat milk, because they can affect consistency.

TIP

● If you make pudding from scratch—and its flavor is so vastly superior to that from mixes—be sure to follow instructions to the letter about adding eggs. They must be added carefully so their proteins don't coagulate.

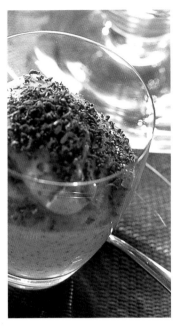

If made with good-quality ingredients, chocolate pudding is a flavorsome treat.

WHAT'S IN IT?

These desserts usually include milk or cream, eggs, and sugar, and often cornstarch or tapioca to thicken and add body.

STYLE 5 oz, or ½ cup	CALORIES	CHOLESTEROL mg	SODIUM mg	TOTAL FAT g
Chocolate pudding, homemade, with skim milk	175	55	225	3
Chocolate pudding, instant, made with whole milk	163	16	417	4.6
Rice pudding	231	1.4	121	10.7
Banana pudding	180	0	278	5.1
Flan (3½ oz)	113	12	112	3

WHAT'S THE BEST?

● The milk and eggs in puddings supply good amounts of protein and calcium. One half-cup can provide about 200mg, or about 20 percent of the recommended daily amount, of calcium.

● Homemade. Packaged puddings are high in sodium and include a lot of stabilizers, as well as powdered eggs and powdered milk. Wouldn't you rather spend five minutes more to have something really wonderful?

WHAT'S NOT SO GOOD?

● Flan, or caramel custard. Recipes for this dessert vary, but some include as many as a dozen egg yolks and all are very high in sugar.

● Big portions. Although puddings can supply 10–20 percent of the calcium requirement, they're still dessert.

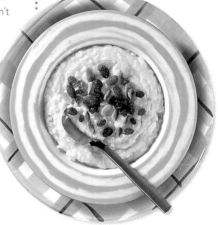

Make your own rice pudding for a dessert that's high in calcium and low in cholesterol.

SATURATED FAT g	PROTEIN g	CARBOHYDRATE g	FIBER g	SUGARS g	GI
1	8	35	tr	NA	NA
2.6	5	27	1.5	NA	NA
1.7	3	31	0.1	NA	NA
0.8	3.4	30	0.1	NA	NA
1.8	3	19	0	NA	H

CHOLATE

● ●

CAN BE HEART-HEALTHY

*I*t's a stretch to call chocolate health food, but it's not as bad for you as you might think.

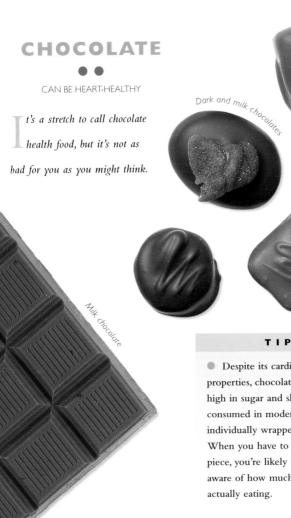

Dark and milk chocolates

Milk chocolate

TIP

● Despite its cardio-protective properties, chocolate is still high in sugar and should be consumed in moderation. Buy individually wrapped chocolates. When you have to unwrap each piece, you're likely to be more aware of how much you're actually eating.

STYLE 1 oz	CALORIES	CHOLESTEROL mg	SODIUM mg	TOTAL FAT g
Semisweet chocolate	136	0	3	8.5
Milk chocolate	144	6	23	8.6
White chocolate	153	6	25	9
Chocolate fudge (1 piece)	70	3	10	1.8

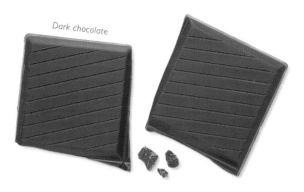

Dark chocolate

WHAT'S IN IT?

Chocolate contains flavonoids that are similar to the cholesterol-lowering compounds in red wine. It also provides some iron; milk chocolate supplies some calcium.

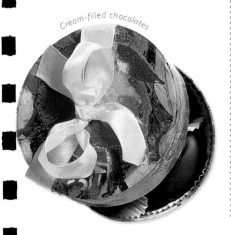

Cream-filled chocolates

WHAT'S THE BEST?

● Dark chocolate, such as bittersweet and semisweet, is highest in antioxidant flavonoids.

● The primary fat in dark chocolate is called stearic acid. It is a type of saturated fat, but it acts like a monounsaturated fat in the body and doesn't raise cholesterol levels.

WHAT'S NOT SO GOOD?

● White chocolate. Technically not a chocolate (it contains no chocolate liquor), it's made primarily of sugar and cocoa butter. It has none of the health benefits attributable to chocolate.

To get the most of chocolate's benefits, opt for solid, not cream- or fruit-filled ones.

SATURATED FAT g	PROTEIN g	CARBOHYDRATE g	FIBER g	SUGARS g	GI
5	1	18	1.7	16	L
5.2	2	17	1	NA	L
5.5	2	17	0	17	NA
1	0.4	13	0.3	NA	NA

CANDIES

●

NOT HEALTHFUL

Unlike chocolate, which has some health benefits, chewy candy and hard candy have little to recommend them. If you want a fruit-flavored treat, grab a real piece of fruit instead.

TIP

● Butterscotch, peanut brittle, and caramels—at least good ones—will never proclaim they are cholesterol-free. That's because high-quality ones are made with butter, and it contains cholesterol.

WHAT'S IN IT?

Most of these candies are heavy on the sugar. Depending on the candy and the recipe, they can include gelatin as a thickener, fat, and flavorings.

Gummy bears

STYLE 1 oz	CALORIES	CHOLESTEROL mg	SODIUM mg	TOTAL FAT g
Butterscotch rounds	111	3	111	0.9
Gummy bears (10)	85	0	10	0
Gumdrops (10)	139	0	16	0
Jelly beans	103	0	7	0.1
Marshmallows	92	0	14	tr
Peanut brittle	139	3	131	5.4
Caramels	108	2	70	2.3
Strawberry licorice	99	0	82	0.7

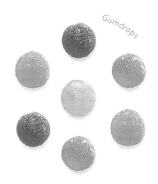

Gumdrops

WHAT'S THE BEST?

● Small sizes. Don't just grab a bag of these. Look on the label to see what a serving is. Count out the number of pieces, but if you find you're satisfied after the sixth gummy bear, put the rest away.

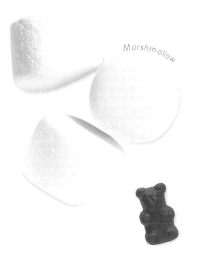

Marshmallow

WHAT'S NOT SO GOOD?

● Don't be impressed by claims of "contains real fruit juice" on packages. Odds are high that it isn't one that's comparatively rich in nutrients but is one that's mild in flavor and not as dense in vitamins and minerals, like grape juice. And odds are higher that only a very small amount of juice is actually used.

● Sticky candies glom onto your teeth, particularly in the crevices and crannies in molars. If you can't brush your teeth right after eating them, at least drink a glass of water to rinse off as much of the sugar as you can.

SATURATED FAT g	PROTEIN g	CARBOHYDRATE g	FIBER g	SUGARS g	GI
0.6	tr	26	0	NA	NA
0	0	22	0	NA	NA
0	0	36	0	NA	NA
tr	0	26	0	NA	H
tr	0.5	23	tr	16	NA
1.3	2	20	0.7	NA	NA
1.9	1	22	0.3	18.6	NA
0	0.7	23	0	11.3	NA

COOKIES AND BARS

●

NOT HEALTHFUL

*I*f you've got a sweet tooth, indulging it with a cookie isn't the best choice, but it isn't the worst, either. Some cookies are low in fat, but even "healthy" ones like oatmeal and peanut butter are still low in nutrients.

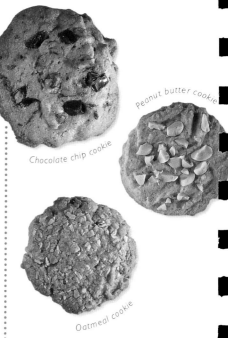

Chocolate chip cookie

Peanut butter cookie

Oatmeal cookie

TIP

 Some people like quantity— one cookie won't do. If you're one of these people, make or buy small cookies. A few little cookies will provide the same calories, fat, and carbohydrate as one larger one.

WHAT'S IN IT?

If you've ever made a batch of cookies, you know that the primary ingredients are refined flour, refined sugar, fat, and eggs. Flavorings like vanilla or spices and mix-ins like oatmeal or chocolate chips vary.

STYLE 1 each	CALORIES	CHOLESTEROL mg	SODIUM mg	TOTAL FAT g
Chocolate chip (2¼-inch)	78	11	55	4.5
Chocolate sandwich cookie with cream filling	47	0	60	2
Peanut butter	95	6	104	4.8
Oatmeal	67	5	90	2.7
Sugar	66	4	69	3.3
Gingersnap	118	0	186	2.8
Brownie (2-inch square)	112	18	82	7
Fig bar	56	0	56	1.2

WHAT'S THE BEST?

● Homemade. Yes, it takes time to make a batch of cookies, but because you don't have to worry about how long they sit on a shelf, yours will be free of unnecessary preservatives.

WHAT'S NOT SO GOOD?

● Shortening and margarine. Whether you make cookies with these fats at home or whether you buy cookies made with these hydrogenated fats, you're getting harmful trans fats with every cookie.

● Fat-free cookies. Often no lower in calories than regular cookies, fat-free cookies are a lot easier to overeat than regular ones. Fat is satisfying and helps to fill you up. Better to grab one or two full-fat cookies than plow through a row of fat-free ones.

Gingerbread man

Butter cookies

SATURATED FAT g	PROTEIN g	CARBOHYDRATE g	FIBER g	SUGARS g	GI
2.3	0.9	9	NA	NA	NA
0.4	0.5	7	0.3	NA	NA
0.9	2	12	NA	NA	NA
0.5	1	10	NA	NA	L
0.7	0.8	8	0.2	NA	NA
0.7	2	22	0.6	NA	NA
1.8	1.5	12	NA	NA	NA
0.2	0.6	11	0.7	NA	NA

CAKES AND PASTRIES

●

HIGH IN SUGAR. CAN BE
HIGH IN TRANS FATS

*Y*ou know they're high in
calories, sugar, fat, and
everything else that you're not
supposed to eat, but the
numbers might
surprise you.

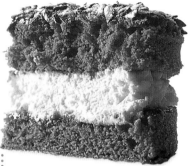

Chocolate cake

Chocolate éclair

WHAT'S IN IT?

Even fruit-based desserts like
pineapple upside-down cake and
apple or berry pie are high in added
sugar; with the exception of angel food
cake, most desserts are high in fat; all
are high in refined flours. Consider
skipping dessert for a few days, then
have a piece of what you really love.

STYLE	CALORIES	CHOLESTEROL mg	SODIUM mg	TOTAL FAT g
Cake (1/12 of an 8-, 9-, or 10-inch cake)				
Angel food (10-inch)	129	0	255	0.2
Chocolate, w/o frosting (9-inch)	340	55	299	14.3
Pineapple upside-down (1/9 of 8-inch square)	367	25	367	13.9
Yellow, w/o frosting (8-inch)	245	37	233	9.9
Chocolate frosting (2 tbsp)	163	0	75	7.2
Cheesecake	321	55	207	22.5
Pie and pastry (1/8 of 9-inch dessert)				
Apple pie	411	0	327	19
Banana cream pie	387	73	346	19.6
Lemon meringue pie	362	67	307	16.4
Pecan pie	503	106	320	27
Pumpkin pie	316	65	349	14.4
Chocolate-covered éclair (approx 5 x 2 x 2 inches)	262	127	337	15.7

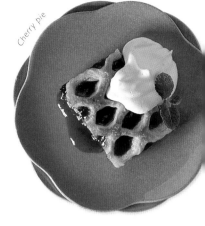

Cherry pie

WHAT'S THE BEST?

● Go for the pumpkin pie. It's lower in calories, fat, and carbs than most of the other alternatives, and it provides about 12,000 IU of vitamin A. That's about the amount in a 1/3 cup of cooked carrots, though a slice of the pie has ten times more calories than the carrots do.

WHAT'S NOT SO GOOD?

● Shortening. Look for piecrust recipes that use vegetable oil, or use lard. to Believe it or not, this much-maligned fat is lower in trans fats than shortening and lower in cholesterol and saturated fats than butter, and it makes remarkably tender, flaky pie crusts.

SATURATED FAT g	PROTEIN g	CARBOHYDRATE g	FIBER g	SUGARS g	GI
tr	3	29	0.1	NA	NA
5.2	5	51	1.5	NA	NA
3.4	4	58	0.9	NA	NA
2.7	4	36	0.5		
2.3	0.5	26	0.4	24	NA
9.9	6	26	0.4	NA	NA
4.7	4	58	NA	NA	NA
5.4	6	47	1	NA	NA
4	5	50	NA	NA	NA
4.9	6	64	NA	NA	NA
4.9	7	41	NA	NA	NA
4.1	6	24	0.6	NA	NA

SUGAR, HONEY, JAMS, AND SPREADS

●

NOT HEALTHFUL

*I*f there were a food that had no nutritional value whatsoever, and had the potential to ruin your teeth and maybe even cause diabetes, would you eat 20 teaspoons of it a day?

TIP

● Despite their rich-sounding name, fruit butters are fat-free and, depending on the recipe, can be fairly low in added sugar, too.

WHAT'S IN IT?

Although some forms of sugar—honey, maple syrup, brown sugar, molasses, and jam—contain trace amounts of nutrients, sugar is either entirely or almost entirely simple carbohydrate.

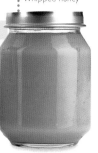
Whipped honey

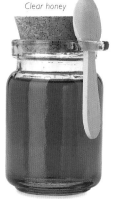
Clear honey

STYLE 1 teaspoon, unless noted	CALORIES	CHOLESTEROL mg	SODIUM mg	TOTAL FAT g
Granulated sugar	16	0	tr	0
Brown sugar (packed)	17	0	2	0
Powdered sugar	10	0	tr	tr
Honey	21	0	0.3	0
Maple syrup (1 tbsp)	52	0	2	tr
Molasses (1 tbsp)	53	0	7	tr
All-fruit spread, strawberry (1 tbsp)	42	0	4	0
Jam, apricot (1 tbsp)	48	0	8	tr
Jam, all other flavors (1 tbsp)	56	0	6	tr
Apple butter (1 tbsp)	29	0	0.7	0

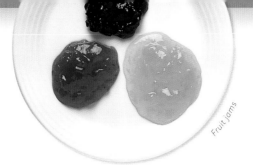
Fruit jams

WHAT'S THE BEST?

● With one exception, this is one category where there really is no best. You might add only one or two spoons of sugar onto your cereal in the morning, and you might not think that you're eating any sugar at lunch or dinner. However, sugar and sweeteners lurk in so many foods (often in the form of high-fructose corn syrup) that it's far easier to eat far more than you think you are.

● Blackstrap molasses. One tablespoon contains 47 calories, 12g of carbohydrate, and 172mg of calcium, as well as other minerals. It has a very pronounced flavor, however—it's not something you'd want to stir into your coffee.

WHAT'S NOT SO GOOD?

● All-fruit spreads and jams. The spreads don't have additional sugar, at least not the white granulated stuff. They're often made with grape juice, which is high in fruit sugar and has few nutrients. Three teaspoons of jam contains 2 1/2 teaspoons of sugar.

● Honey. Some tout it as a cure-all, and it does contain antioxidants, but you'd have to eat an awful lot of honey to get the any benefits. Honey can contain small amounts of botulism spores and should never be given to children under 1 year old. Babies don't produce digestive acids in sufficient amounts to render the spores harmless, though older children and adults do.

SATURATED FAT g	PROTEIN g	CARBOHYDRATE g	FIBER g	SUGARS g	GI
0	0	4.2	0	4.2	M
0	0	4.5	0	4	NA
0	0	2.5	0	2	NA
0	tr	5.8	tr	5	H
0	0	13.4	0	12.7	NA
0	0	13.8	0	12	NA
0	0.1	10	0	7.6	NA
0	0.1	13	0.2	9	NA
0	tr	13.8	0.2	9.7	NA
0	tr	7	0.2	6	NA

SAUCES AND CONDIMENTS

●

HIGH IN SODIUM.
CAN BE HIGH IN SUGAR

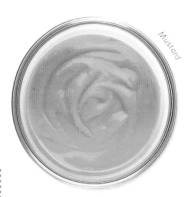

Mustard

These are easy ways to add flavor. They're often high in sugar and sodium, but they're typically used in small amounts.

TIP

● Ketchup is squirted out of a bottle, mayonnaise and mustard are often scooped out of the jar. Measure a serving, then spoon that amount onto your plate or food and compare how this amount looks to what you typically use.

WHAT'S IN IT?

Ketchup contains mostly tomatoes by weight, but it's still a far cry from a tomato nutritionally. A tablespoon of ketchup supplies only 2mg vitamin C and 152 IU vitamin A—less than what is in one tomato wedge.

Mayonnaise

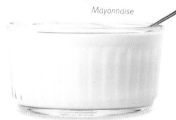

STYLE 1 tablespoon	CALORIES	CHOLESTEROL mg	SODIUM mg	TOTAL FAT g
Ketchup	16	0	178	tr
Mustard (1 tsp)	3	0	56	0.2
Mayonnaise	100	5	80	11
Light mayo	50	5	120	4.9
Sweet pickle relish	20	0	122	tr
Barbecue sauce	12	0	127	0.3
Cheese sauce	30	6	74	2.2
Soy sauce	8	0	914	tr
Taco sauce, red	7	0	105	tr
Pesto	75	0	135	7.1
Italian dressing	69	0	116	7.1
Blue cheese dressing	76	3	164	7.8

Homemade dressings

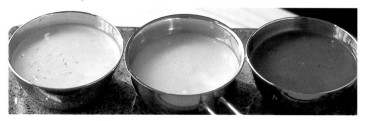

WHAT'S THE BEST?

● Vegetable-based condiments. Pesto and tapenade (a paste made of olives) tend to be high in fat, but olives or olive oil are primary ingredients, so they're more healthful than sugary sauces.

● Homemade dressings. It takes about a minute to whip up a salad dressing, and one that's freshly made tastes vastly better than storebought. Plus you can avoid unnecessary sweeteners and stabilizers, and you know the quality of the ingredients.

WHAT'S NOT SO GOOD?

● Large amounts. One packet of ketchup from a fast-food restaurant is slightly more than 1 teaspoon. After you've ripped open a few packets it's easy to lose track of how much you're really eating.

● Mayonnaise-based sauces. Tartar sauce and aïoli share mayo's high-fat, high-calorie profile and are best eaten sparingly. Because they're higher in flavor, though, a little of them may go farther than a small amount of mayonnaise.

SATURATED FAT g	PROTEIN g	CARBOHYDRATE g	FIBER g	SUGARS g	GI
0	0.2	4	0.2	4	NA
tr	0.2	0.4	0.2	0	NA
1.5	0	0	0	0	NA
0.8	tr	1.3	tr	0.6	NA
tr	tr	5	0.2	4	NA
tr	0.3	2	0.2	2	NA
1.2	2	0.6	tr	NA	NA
0	0.8	1.4	0.1	0	NA
0	0.2	1.3	tr	1	NA
NA	3	1	0.5	NA	NA
1	0.1	1.5	0	NA	NA
1.5	0.7	1.1	0	NA	NA

BEER AND WINE

● ●

CAN BE HEART-HEALTHY

*B*eer and wine may play a role *in protecting your health, but this is one category where more is not a good thing.*

WHAT'S IN IT?

Alcohol contains 7 calories per gram (compared to 9 calories per gram of fat and 4 calories per gram of protein or of carbohydrate). Beer provides some B vitamins and wine contains small amounts of iron, but neither beverage supplies them in amounts to provide significant nutritional benefits.

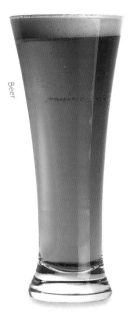

Beer

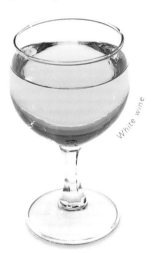

White wine

STYLE 12-oz serving	CALORIES	CHOLESTEROL mg	SODIUM mg	TOTAL FAT g
Light beer	99	0	11	0
Low-carb beer	95	0	NA	0
Lager beer	146	0	18	0
Dry red wine (5 oz)	107	0	7	0
Dry white wine (5 oz)	100	0	7	0

WHAT'S THE BEST?

● Red wine contains the highest concentrations of flavonoids, particularly resveratrol, which is found in grape skins. These antioxidants are thought to increase HDL ("good") cholesterol levels and may prevent blood from clotting.

WHAT'S NOT SO GOOD?

● Immoderate drinking. For health benefits, researchers recommend no more than one 12-oz beer, 5 oz of wine, or 1 1/2 oz of liquor per day for women, or twice that per day for men.

TIP

● Unlike food, alcohol isn't digested, it's absorbed into the bloodstream. Eating something with your drink will slow the absorption rate.

Drunk in moderate quantities, red wine does have health-promoting benefits.

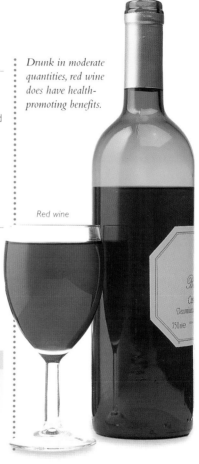

Red wine

SATURATED FAT g	PROTEIN g	CARBOHYDRATE g	FIBER g	SUGARS g	GI
0	0.7	4.6	0	NA	NA
0	0.6	2.6	NA	NA	NA
0	1	13	2	NA	NA
0	0.3	2.4	0	NA	NA
0	0.1	1.1	0	NA	NA

TEA, COFFEE, HOT CHOCOLATE, AND WHIPPED DRINKS

● ●

SOME CAN BE HEART-HEALTHY

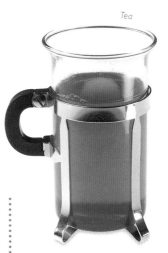

Tea

*T*ea has been linked to an astonishing number of health benefits. The jury's still out on coffee, but some of the latest research indicates that it isn't as harmful as previously thought. Beware of latte and other coffee drinks—they can be loaded with sugar and fat, and have calorie counts to match.

TIP

● Chai is a drink made of tea, spices, milk, and a sweetener. Make your own by steeping spices like cinnamon, cloves, cardamom, nutmeg, ginger root, and peppercorns with loose tea, then straining and adding milk or cream and sweetener.

STYLE 10-oz serving, unless noted	CALORIES	CHOLESTEROL mg	SODIUM mg	TOTAL FAT g
Brewed tea	3	0	9	0
Coffee, black	6	0	6	0
Hot chocolate	240	2	16	.8
Dunkin Donuts Vanilla Chai	230	5	50	8
Coffee Coolatta, made with whole milk (16 oz)	210	15	80	4
Orange Mango Coolatta (16 oz)	270	0	25	0
McDonald's Vanilla Triple Thick Shake (16 oz)	570	65	400	16

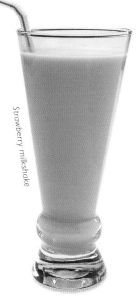

Coffee

Strawberry milkshake

WHAT'S THE BEST?

● Homemade. Restaurant shakes, smoothies, and chai drinks are expensive, and often include chemicals, fruit concentrates, and high-fructose corn syrup. Make these drinks at home and you can use the ingredients you prefer for pennies.

WHAT'S IN IT?

Tea contains catechins, compounds that can reduce the risk of some cancers and boost the immune system. Green tea contains higher concentrations of catechins than black tea does.

WHAT'S NOT SO GOOD?

● Coffee and tea are low in calories and nutrients. Add milk or cream, sugar, and flavored syrups and the numbers skyrocket.

SATURATED FAT g	PROTEIN g	CARBOHYDRATE g	FIBER g	SUGARS g	GI
0	0	.9	0	0	NA
0	tr	1	0	0	NA
.5	1	4	0.3	NA	NA
6	1	40	0	32	NA
2.5	4	42	0	40	NA
0	1	66	2	58	NA
11	14	89	0	76	NA

SODA, WATER, AND SPORT DRINKS

CAN BE HIGH IN SUGAR

If you're really thirsty, then plain old water, rather than high-sugar drinks, is usually the best quencher.

TIP

● Gatorade was developed for the University of Florida Gators football team as an easy way replace electrolytes (minerals necessary for proper metabolic function) and rehydrate. If you work outdoors for hours in weather that borders on jungle-like, sport beverages might be worth your while.

WHAT'S IN IT?

Soda is one of the leading sources of sugar in the diet —a 12-oz can contains 8 or 9 teaspoons; a large soda from a fast-food restaurant contains 24 teaspoons, or a 1/2 cup.

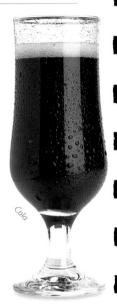

Cola

STYLE 12-oz can, unless noted	CALORIES	CHOLESTEROL mg	SODIUM mg	TOTAL FAT g
Lemon-lime soda	147	0	41	0
Ginger ale	124	0	26	0
Club soda	0	0	75	0
Diet cola	0	0	21	0
Cola	152	0	15	0
Cola (32 oz, large)	403	0	39	0
Cola, (44 oz, super size)	555	0	54	0
Gatorade, all flavors (8 oz)	50	0	110	0
Sobe Orange Carrot Elixir				
8-oz serving	90	0	15	0
20-oz bottle	225	0	38	0

Mineral water

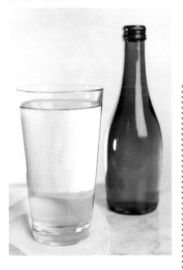

WHAT'S NOT SO GOOD?

● 20-oz bottles. Whether you're buying a soda, a tea beverage, or an herbal elixir, these bottles all have Nutrition Facts based on 8-oz servings—that's 2½ servings per bottle. But do you really stop when you've drunk ²/₅ of the bottle, or do you keep swigging?

● High-fructose corn syrup. An inexpensive sweetener used in just about everything, even in "healthful" beverages. It's just another name for sugar, as a quick look at the carbohydrate and sugars on the Nutrition Facts label bears out.

● Stealth caffeine. You expect it in colas, but it's also in some brands of orange or other citrusy sodas.

WHAT'S THE BEST?

● Mineral water contains small amounts of minerals—12 oz of club soda, for instance, supplies about ¹/₁₀₀ of your calcium requirements for the day—but not enough to supply health benefits beyond still or tap water.

SATURATED FAT g	PROTEIN g	CARBOHYDRATE g	FIBER g	SUGARS g	GI
0	0	38	0	38	H
0	0	32	0	32	H
0	0	0	0	0	L
0	0	tr	0	0	L
0	0	38	0	38	H
0	0	102	0	102	H
0	0	141	0	141	H
0	0	14	0	14	NA
0	0	24	0	24	H
0	0	60	0	60	H

JUICE AND JUICE DRINKS

● ●

CAN BE HEALTHFUL

*I*f it's made of 100 percent juice and it contains all-natural ingredients it has to be good for you— or at least better than soda, right?

TIP

● Dilute juice with seltzer for a refreshing alternative to soda. Try some of the flavored seltzers—orange seltzer with cranberry juice, for instance, or raspberry seltzer with orange or white grape juice.

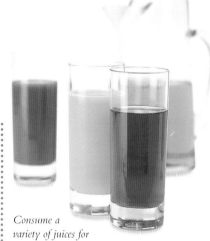

Consume a variety of juices for the most nutrients—but limit the amounts you drink.

WHAT'S IN IT?

As with the foods they come from, juices contain different amounts of vitamins (they're usually high in C and A), and they can be high in sugars.

STYLE 8-oz	CALORIES	CHOLESTEROL mg	SODIUM mg	TOTAL FAT g
Apple, unsweetened	117	0	7	0.3
Orange, fresh	112	0	2	0.5
Cranberry, unsweetened	116	0	5	0.3
Carrot	94	0	68	0.4
Grape, unsweetened	154	0	8	0.2
Grapefruit, white	96	0	2	0.2
Grapefruit, pink	96	0	2	0.2
Fruit punch	124	0	12	0.5
Peach nectar	134	0	17	tr
Vegetable juice cocktail	46	0	653	0.2
Cranberry juice cocktail	144	0	5	0.3
Pineapple juice, unsweetened	140	0	3	0.2
Prune, unsweetened	182	0	10	tr
Tomato juice	41	0	24	0.1

WHAT'S THE BEST?

⬤ Vegetable juices tend to be higher in fiber and lower in sugars than fruit juices. Blend apple with carrot or orange with carrot (or mix all three) to boost nutrients.

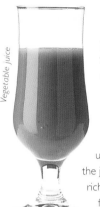

Vegetable juice

⬤ Most juices contain the same phytochemicals as the foods they come from, but not all. If most of the compounds are in the peel and only the pulp is used to make juice, the juice won't be as rich a source as the fruit will be.

WHAT'S NOT SO GOOD?

⬤ As far as your body's concerned, sugar—whether fructose (fruit sugar) or sucrose (refined white table sugar)—is sugar. Juices boast vitamins, minerals and antioxidants that sodas don't, but juices can be fairly high in calories, and they're lower in fiber than the fruit they come from. Consume them in moderation.

⬤ Fiber levels. Compare the amounts in the chart below to the amounts in the charts in the fruits and vegetable chapter.

⬤ Juice blends. Read ingredient lists for exotic and blended juices. Odds are high that the mango-papaya 100 percent juice drink contains more apple or grape juice than mango or papaya.

SATURATED FAT g	PROTEIN g	CARBOHYDRATE g	FIBER g	SUGARS g	GI
tr	0.1	29	0.2	27	NA
tr	2	26	0.5	20	NA
tr	1	31	0.3	31	NA
tr	2	22	1.9	9	NA
tr	1	38	0.2	38	NA
tr	1	23	0.3	22	NA
tr	1	23	NA	NA	NA
tr	0.2	30	0.2	NA	NA
tr	0.7	35	1.5	33	NA
tr	2	11	0.3	34	NA
tr	0	36	0.3	34	NA
tr	0.8	34	0.5	34	NA
tr	2	45	2.6	42	NA
tr	2	10	1	9	NA

Further Reading

Looking for more information? The next four pages contain alphabetical lists of books and Web sites that you may find helpful. Many of the Web sites are affiliated with newsletters or magazines, if you prefer your information on paper rather than online.

American Dietetic Association Complete Food and Nutrition Guide
ROBERTA DUYFF
(Wiley, 2002)
Clear explanations of the fundamentals of nutrition, with additional sections for children, women, the elderly, and vegetarians.

Atkins for Life
DR. ROBERT C. ATKINS
(St. Martin's Press, 2003)
Information on following a controlled-carbohydrate eating plan and making it a way of life rather than a "diet." Includes recipes.

Bowes & Church's Food Values of Portions Commonly Used (17th ed.)
JEAN A.T. PENNINGTON
(Lippincott-Raven Publishers, 1998)
Nutrient data for thousands of foods, based on an older version of the USDA's Database for Standard Reference, and on information from food companies, trade associations, and scientific literature.

Cheese Primer
STEVEN JENKINS
(Workman, 1996)
Everything you need or want to know to choose and enjoy the best, most flavorful cheeses.

The Complete Book of Food Counts
CORINNE T. NETZER
(Dell, 2000)
Alphabetical listing of nutrient data for packaged foods and fast-food items.

The Complete Meat Cookbook
BRUCE AIDELLS and DENIS KELLY
(Chapters, 1998)
Excellent information on every sort of meat, with sophisticated, authoritative recipes.

The Food Lover's Companion (3rd ed.)
SHARON TYLER HERBST
(Barron's Educational Series, 2001)
Definitions and explanations of nearly 6,000 culinary terms.
It's also available online at:
eat.epicurious.com/dictionary/food

The Good Fat, Bad Fat Counter
SHEILA BUFF
(St. Martin's Press, 2000)
If you're at all confused about trans fats, omega-3s, and omega-6s, this little book explains them—and more—clearly and accessibly.

Great Fish, Quick
LESLIE REVSIN
(Doubleday, 1997—out of print)
If you're interested in eating more
fish but aren't sure how to cook
it, this is a great book, full of
delicious recipes that can be on
the table in 45 minutes or less.

*The Kitchen Survival Guide: A
Hand-Holding Kitchen Primer with
130 Recipes to Get You Started*
LORA BRODY
(William Morrow, 1992)
Basic, rock-solid information for
kitchen neophytes about cooking
and eating nutritiously. Plus
it's hilarious.

Learning to Cook
MARION CUNNINGHAM
(Random House, 1999)
Not always low-fat or low-carb,
but if you need to learn cooking
fundamentals and want clearly
explained recipes, this is an
excellent resource.

*The NutriBase Guide to Fast-Food
Nutrition*
(Avery, 2001)
Part of a series that provides
nutrient data for a variety of foods
and food groups; this includes
information about food from more
than 65 restaurants.

The Nutrition Bible
JEAN ANDERSON, M.S. and
BARBARA DESKINS, PH.D., R.D.
(William Morrow, 1995)
No longer cutting-edge, but
solid information nonetheless.
Includes recipes.

Stop the Clock! Cooking
CHERYL FORBERG, R.D.
(Avery, 2003)
If you're wondering what
antioxidants are and why they're
important, you'll be hard pressed
to find a clearer explanation
than the first chapter.

Vegetables from Amaranth to Zucchini
ELIZABETH SCHNEIDER
(William Morrow, 2001)
With this in your library, you'll
no longer have to walk past the
jicama or the kohlrabi at the
market because you don't know
what to do with them.

Wellness Foods A to Z
SHELDON MARGEN, M.D., and
the Editors of the University of
California, Berkeley Wellness Letter
(Rebus, 2002)
An A to Z encyclopedia of
nutrition information and food facts.

Useful Web Sites

When you search for information on the Internet, pay careful attention to the source. The site of a major hospital or a doctor affiliated with one is likely to be more reliable than one touting Bahama Bob's Cure-All Energy Pills. URLs that end with ".org" or ".gov" or ".edu" are often reputable, but that isn't to say that addresses with a ".com" aren't trustworthy. If the news sounds too good to be true, it probably is.
Even if the information you find is from a reliable source, run it past your doctor or healthcare practitioner—it may not be right for you.

The Web site for the American Heart Association
www.americanheart.org

The Web site for Atkins Nutritionals, Inc.
www.atkins.com

The University of California's Wellness Newsletter has a subscriber's-only section where archives are available, but its all-access areas contain some useful information, too.
www.berkeleywellness.com

Online search for Glycemic Index of foods, from Australia's University of Sydney
www.calvin.biochem.usyd.edu.au/GIDB/searchD3.htm

The Web site for the American Cancer Society
www.cancer.org

The Web site for the Centers for Disease Control and Prevention
www.cdc.gov

The Web site for the Center for Science in the Public Interest, a consumer watchdog group
www.cspi.org

Rick Mendosa's International Table of Glycemic Index and Glycemic Load Values
http://diabetes.about.com/library/mendosagi/ngilists.htm

Dole Foods' Five-a-Day Web site explains the importance of fruits and vegetables.
www.dole5aday.com

The Web site for the American Dietetic Association
www.eatright.org

A popular online community for weight loss.
www.ediets.com

Harvard University has an extensive list of publications; its online newsletters can be found at:
www.health.Harvard.edu

The Mayo Clinic's extensive consumer Web site: **www.mayoclinic.com**

Rick Mendosa's Glycemic Values of Common American Foods
www.mendosa.com/common_foods.htm

The main entry page for the UDSA's Nutrient Data Laboratory database for Food Composition
www.nal.usda.gov/fnic/foodcomp

The USDA's Food and Nutrition Information Center is similar to the Food Composition main entry page, but the information is arranged differently and it has links to other sites.
www.nal.usda.gov/fnic/etext/000020.html

If you want to check the USDA's database for a specific food, this link takes you directly to the search page.
www.nal.usda.gov/fnic/cgi-bin/nut_search.pl

Tufts University's Nutrition Navigator is a clearinghouse for different Web sites in a variety of medical categories.
www.navigator.tufts.edu

Lists of links to other organizations like the National Cancer Institute; the National Heart, Lung, & Blood Institute.
www.nih.gov/icd

Looking for a specific study? Here's the Web site for the National Institutes of Health and the U.S. National Library of Medicine.
www.nlm.nih.gov/medlineplus/
OR
www.ncbi.nlm.nih.gov/PubMed

The same information as the USDA's, presented in a more user-friendly format.
www.nutritiondata.com

Produce Information and Seasonal Calendar
www.nutritiouslygourmet.com/html/produce.html

Another popular online community for weight loss.
www.weightwatchers.com

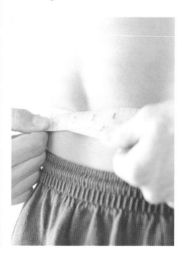

Index

Acknowledgments

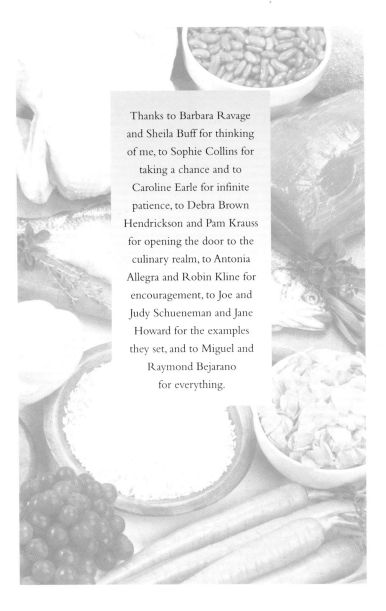

Thanks to Barbara Ravage and Sheila Buff for thinking of me, to Sophie Collins for taking a chance and to Caroline Earle for infinite patience, to Debra Brown Hendrickson and Pam Krauss for opening the door to the culinary realm, to Antonia Allegra and Robin Kline for encouragement, to Joe and Judy Schueneman and Jane Howard for the examples they set, and to Miguel and Raymond Bejarano for everything.